DATE DUE			

30408000001120

613
FOR

Ford, Jean.

Right on schedule! :
a teen's guide to
growth and
development

Woodland High School
Henry County Public Schools

752467 02495   52207A   0022

RIGHT ON SCHEDULE!

A Teen's Guide to Growth and Development

The Science of Health:
Youth and Well-Being

RIGHT ON SCHEDULE!

A Teen's Guide to Growth and Development

by Jean Ford

Mason Crest Publishers

Philadelphia

Mason Crest Publishers Inc.
370 Reed Road, Broomall, Pennsylvania 19008
(866) MCP-BOOK (toll free)
www.masoncrest.com

13 12 11 10 09 08 07 06   10 9 8 7 6 5 4 3

Library of Congress Cataloging-in-Publication Data

Ford, Jean.
  Right on schedule! : a teen's guide to growth and development / by Jean Ford.
     p. cm.
  Includes bibliographical references and index.
        ISBN 1-59084-850-0
        ISBN 1-59084-840-3 (series)
1. Teenagers—Health and hygiene. 2. Adolescence. 3. Adolescent psychology. I. Title.
  RJ141.F67 2004
  613'.0433—dc22
                    2004006297

Designed and produced by Harding House Publishing Service, Vestal, NY 13850.
www.hardinghousepages.com
Cover design by Benjamin Stewart.
Printed and bound in Malaysia.

INTRODUCTION

by Dr. Sara Forman

You're not a little kid anymore. When you look in the mirror, you probably see a new person, someone who's taller, bigger, with a face that's starting to look more like an adult's than a child's. And the changes you're experiencing on the inside may be even more intense than the ones you see in the mirror. Your emotions are changing, your attitudes are changing, and even the way you think is changing. Your friends are probably more important to you than they used to be, and you no longer expect your parents to make all your decisions for you. You may be asking more questions and posing more challenges to the adults in your life. You might experiment with new identities—new ways of dressing, hairstyles, ways of talking—as you try to determine just who you really are. Your body is maturing sexually, giving you a whole new set of confusing and exciting feelings. Sorting out what is right and wrong for you may seem overwhelming.

Growth and development during adolescence is a multifaceted process involving every aspect of you being. It all happens so fast that it can be confusing an distressing. But this stage of your life is entirely norma Every adult in your life made it through adolescence and you will too.

But what exactly is adolescence? According to the American Heritage Dictionary, adolescence is "the period of physical and psychological development from the onset of puberty to maturity." What does this really mean?

In essence, adolescence is the time in our lives when the needs of childhood give way to the responsibilities of adulthood. According to psychologist Erik Erikson, these years are a time of separation and individuation. In other words, you are separating from your parents, becoming an individual in your own right. These are the years when you begin to make decisions on your own. You are becoming more self-reliant and less dependent on family members.

When medical professionals look at what's happening physically—what they refer to as the biological model—they define the teen years as a period of hormonal transformation toward sexual maturity, as well as a time of peak growth, second only to the growth during the months of infancy. This physical transformation from childhood to adulthood takes place under the influence of society's norms and social pressures; at the same time your body is changing, the people around you are expecting new things from you. This is what makes adolescence such a unique and challenging time.

Being a teenager in North America today is exciting yet stressful. For those who work with teens, whether by parenting them, educating them, or providing services to them, adolescence can be challenging as well. Youth are struggling with many messages from society and the media about how they should behave and who they should be. "Am I normal?" and "How do I fit in?" are often questions with which teens wrestle. They are facing decisions about their health such as how to take care of their bodies, whether to use drugs and alcohol, or whether to have sex.

This series of books on adolescents' health issues provides teens, their parents, their teachers, and all those who work with them accurate information and the tools to keep them safe and healthy. The topics include information about:

- normal growth
- social pressures
- emotional issues
- specific diseases to which adolescents are prone
- stressors facing youth today
- sexuality

The series is a dynamic set of books, which can be shared by youth and the adults who care for them. By providing this information to educate in these areas, these books will help build a foundation for readers so they can begin to work on improving the health and well-being of youth today.

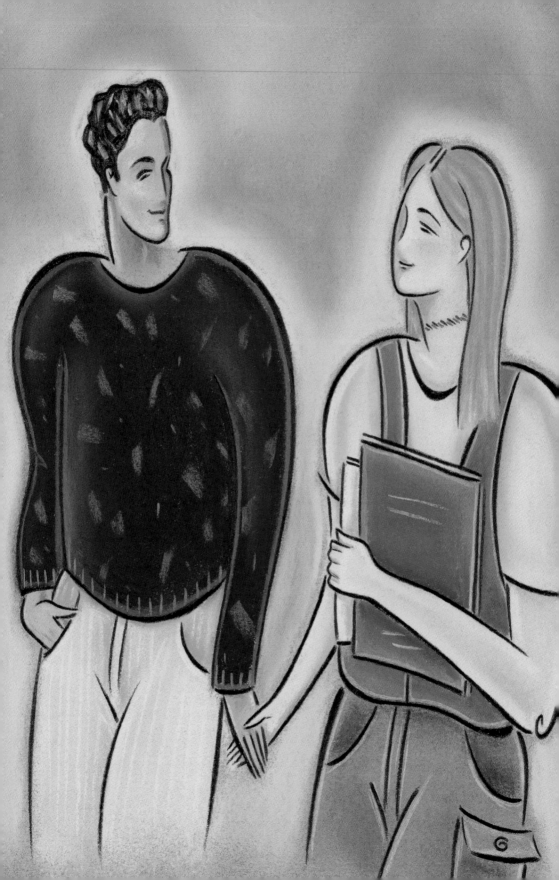

1
EXTREME DESIGN:
The One and Only You

Monica taps a pencil nervously on her desk. The kids here look so different from her private school! All kinds of faces surround her: freckled faces tickled with curls; mocha faces gripped in braids; tan faces draped in silk; and porcelain faces cupped by ebony. Make-up, spikes, perms, piercings . . . every face is unique, even exotic. Monica looks forward to getting to know the people behind the faces, but she has to admit she's scared. *They all seem so cool I hope someone will like me . . .*

Jon looks older than sixteen. His mature good looks, muscular build, and expensive clothes are definite advantages, but this year he also happens to be the "new" kid. As he makes his way to his locker, all kinds of teens clutter the view: Goths, jocks, and druggies; the dyed, tattooed, and pierced; the plain and the "perfect"; the overdeveloped and underdeveloped; the hairy, bearded, bald, and baby-faced. Jon sighs. *What a bunch of losers. Why did Dad have to move here?*

Two typical high schools. Two new students. Two opposite reactions.

Monica thinks she's inferior, even unlikable, because she sees herself as plain, less interesting than the other kids. She observes their physical diversity self-consciously, yet remains optimistic. Despite her insecurities, she longs to fit in.

Jon, in turn, is aloof, arrogant and judgmental. He thinks he's superior because of his appearance, as if he had any say in it. His M.O. is to keep his distance from these "losers." He wouldn't be caught dead with most of them. (But does he even know them?)

Have you ever thought like Monica or Jon? Have you ever felt awkward or ashamed about a part of your body, particularly when you compared yourself with others? How about superior? Chances are you have. As different as Monica's and Jon's reactions are, their feelings permeate high school hallways across the continent, including yours.

Maybe you've witnessed friends call other teens nasty names based on appearances. Maybe you've done that yourself, or been on the receiving end of such insults. Teens gravitate toward those who are similar to them, and they tend to make fun of or avoid those who aren't. It's common, unfair, and often sad, but such choices are usually based on insecurity, fear, or ignorance.

"Help! I'm being held prisoner by my heredity and environment!"

—Dennis Allen

Have you ever heard anyone comment, "It's in the **genes**?" They were probably speaking of a talent or physical trait. What we're good at, what we look like, and how we grow *is* "in the genes." Genes are passed down to us from our parents. No one has a choice in the matter. Family circumstance, lifestyles, religious beliefs, neighborhoods, and cultures, however, can impact our abilities and appearance. By now, you may be thinking, *Help! I'm being held prisoner by my heredity and environment!*

Why, then, do young people condemn, praise, boast, or apologize for things over which no kid has control? With the exception of exercise, diet, hygiene, and cosmetics, we have little to do with how we look and the rate at which we mature. Genes determine every trait. No diet will lengthen my neck or broaden my shoulders. No exercise will make me five-feet-seven or my turn hair fine and straight. Some teens are just more bony, others more muscular; some will be busty and others more flat-chested. And most will be perfectly normal.

The Blueprint: Our Genetic Heritage

Genes are blueprints for development. They determine human characteristics such as height, body type, hair and eye color, and propensities toward specific abilities. To fully understand how they work, let's back up.

Every living thing is made up of cells. Each cell contains a substance called DNA (deoxyribonucleic acid). (You might have heard of DNA on crime shows or in criminal investigations. It's often used to identify "who-dunit" because no two people share exactly the same DNA arrangements.) DNA contains chemicals strung in distinct patterns on coiled strands inside each cell. These patterns contain codes for manufacturing the proteins that enable your body to function. The DNA, with all these patterns, wraps together to form structures called chromosomes. Genes carry instructions for development on these chromosomes (for example, instructions for producing eye pigment.)

Science Fiction and Genetics

- Did you know that the idea of manipulating genes to perfect humanity has been around since the early 1900s? Read A. Huxley's novel *Brave New World*, written in 1927. (See if any of his predictions come true!)
- Even Hollywood tackles issues surrounding genetic manipulation. Check out these classic sci-fi thrillers: *Strange New World* (1975), *The Boys from Brazil* (1978), or *Gattaca* (1997).

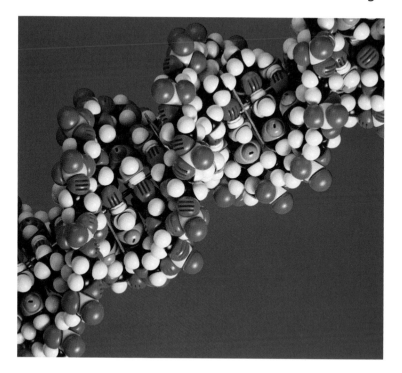

A model of a strand of DNA.

Most human cells have twenty-three pairs of gene-carrying chromosomes, or forty-six total. Because sperm and egg cells each have only twenty-three unpaired chromosomes, every human receives half of his or her chromosomes from each parent at conception. And because each parent provides one chromosome for each pair, you receive two of every gene (two hair, two eye, etc.). Some resulting physical characteristics require only a single gene, while others require two of the same or a combination of two different genes. For example, blue eyes require two blue genes since they are weaker (or *recessive*) genes. Brown eyes can result from either two

15

brown genes or one blue combined with one brown since brown is a stronger (or ***dominant***) gene.

Genes determine color, body type, and growth rate long before we're even born, and every person ends up with approximately 30,000 different genes! The number of potential combinations is almost endless. No wonder we're all different!

To compare ourselves to others—or others to us—is obviously pointless. More important, to feel inferior or superior based on appearance reveals a basic ignorance of human development: it's out of our control. Genes alone don't grant us bragging or berating rights.

No two teens are exactly alike. No height or body shape is perfect or "the standard." You are uniquely and wonderfully you. You will grow as you were genetically wired to grow, and so will every other person you encounter. No one is better or worse, merely different.

Boning Up on Bones

- The human body has 206 living bones.
- Bones are alive!
- Forty to 60 percent of bone mass is built during adolescence.
- Bones are continually "building up" and "breaking down" through a process called remodeling.
- "Breakdown" gradually outpaces "buildup" as we age, and bones become more brittle.
- Both males and females reach peak bone mass by age thirty.

GROWING EVERY DAY: GROWTH CHARTS

Amanda and Katie are both fourteen. They're best friends. They share neighborhood, music and clothing tastes, friends, and even their birth date. But that's where the similarities end. Amanda hit her growth spurt at twelve. Now, at five-feet, six-inches, she looks nearly the woman she will eventually be. Katie, meanwhile, is only five feet tall and still looks more like the child she'd prefer to leave behind: no hips, no boobs, and plenty of "baby fat." Both of them are in the ninth grade. How can they look so different?

By the same token, Ron and Mike are both sophomores, both fifteen, and both wrestlers. Five-foot-six, wiry, and baby-faced, Mike wrestles in the 119-pound class. On the other hand, Ron is six-one, and he's thick and muscular; he wrestles at 189. The pair could be stand-ins for man David and boy Goliath. How can this be?

Teens grow with more diversity than any other age group. To that end, medical experts have designed charts that visually represent the broad range of normal growth that can occur during these years. These charts, developed by the National Center for Health Statistics (NCHS) in collaboration with the National Center for Chronic Disease Prevention (NCCDC), determine how you size up to most teens (of your gender) in height and weight. First find your height and age on the line graph marked "STATURE." Follow these separate lines to where the two lines meet. The point at which they intersect indicates the percentile in which you fall height-wise compared to all teens your age and gender. If, for example, the lines

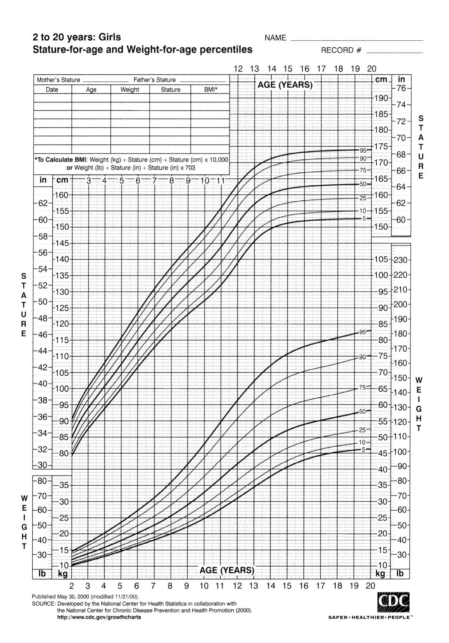

2 to 20 years: Girls
Stature-for-age and Weight-for-age percentiles

NAME _____

RECORD # _____

*To Calculate BMI: Weight (kg) ÷ Stature (cm) ÷ Stature (cm) x 10,000
or Weight (lb) ÷ Stature (in) ÷ Stature (in) x 703

Published May 30, 2000 (modified 11/21/00).
SOURCE: Developed by the National Center for Health Statistics in collaboration with
the National Center for Chronic Disease Prevention and Health Promotion (2000).
http://www.cdc.gov/growthcharts

SAFER·HEALTHIER·PEOPLE™

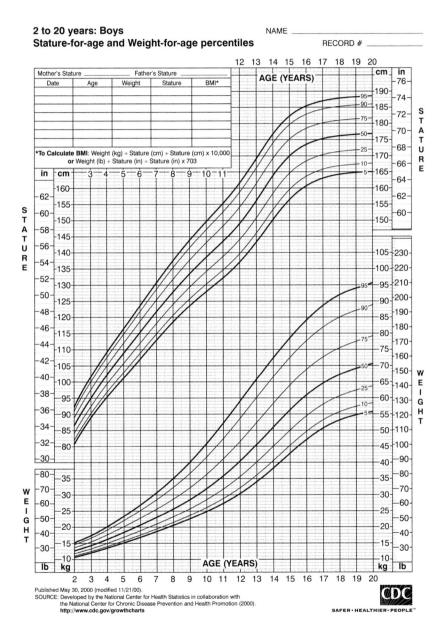

2 to 20 years: Boys
Stature-for-age and Weight-for-age percentiles

NAME _____

RECORD # _____

*To Calculate BMI: Weight (kg) ÷ Stature (cm) ÷ Stature (cm) x 10,000
or Weight (lb) ÷ Stature (in) ÷ Stature (in) x 703

Published May 30, 2000 (modified 11/21/00).
SOURCE: Developed by the National Center for Health Statistics in collaboration with
the National Center for Chronic Disease Prevention and Health Promotion (2000).
http://www.cdc.gov/growthcharts

SAFER · HEALTHIER · PEOPLE™

19

for height and age meet nearest the curved line marked "60," then you're taller than 60 percent of teens the same age and sex, and shorter than 40 percent. That means in a group of a hundred random teens your age and gender, odds are that you'll be taller than sixty of them and shorter than forty of them.

Next, follow the same procedure using the line graph marked "WEIGHT." Find the lines for your weight and age. Where they intersect tells you in what percentile you fall weight-wise compared to other teens. For example, if your weight and age lines intersect nearest the curved line marked "10," then you weigh more than 10 percent of like teens your age, and less than 90 percent. (This percentage does not indicate if your weight is healthy, just how it compares to others in the same age bracket.)

According to these charts, two healthy teens of like gender and age can vary in height by as much as ten inches. Perfectly normal teens of like height can vary in weight by as much as ninety pounds. The key is knowing whether your height-to-weight ratio is good. That presents a problem. How *can* you know if you're maintaining a healthy weight for your height? Again, the NCHS in cooperation with the CDC created a chart and line graph based on calculating your BMI (body mass index).

To find out your BMI, use either of the following equations:

Weight (in kilograms) ÷ height (in meters, squared) = Your BMI

Weight (in pounds) ÷ Height (in inches, squared) x 703 = Your BMI

Here's an example: If you are five feet, six inches tall, and you weigh 165 pounds, turn to page 24 to see what your equation will look like.

2 to 20 years: Girls
Body mass index-for-age percentiles

NAME _____

RECORD # _____

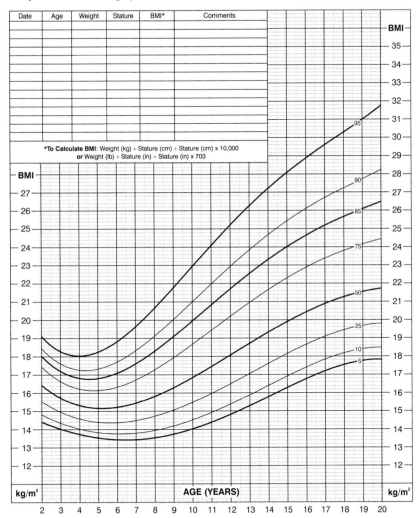

Date	Age	Weight	Stature	BMI*	Comments

*To Calculate BMI: Weight (kg) ÷ Stature (cm) ÷ Stature (cm) x 10,000
or Weight (lb) ÷ Stature (in) ÷ Stature (in) x 703

BMI

AGE (YEARS)

kg/m²

Published May 30, 2000 (modified 10/16/00).
SOURCE: Developed by the National Center for Health Statistics in collaboration with
the National Center for Chronic Disease Prevention and Health Promotion (2000).
http://www.cdc.gov/growthcharts

SAFER · HEALTHIER · PEOPLE™

21

Right On Schedule

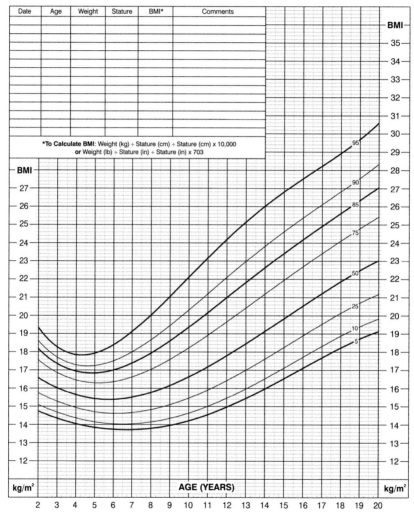

2 to 20 years: Boys
Body mass index-for-age percentiles

NAME _____

RECORD # _____

Date	Age	Weight	Stature	BMI*	Comments

*To Calculate BMI: Weight (kg) ÷ Stature (cm) ÷ Stature (cm) x 10,000
or Weight (lb) ÷ Stature (in) ÷ Stature (in) x 703

AGE (YEARS)

Published May 30, 2000 (modified 10/16/00).
SOURCE: Developed by the National Center for Health Statistics in collaboration with
the National Center for Chronic Disease Prevention and Health Promotion (2000).
http://www.cdc.gov/growthcharts

SAFER·HEALTHIER·PEOPLE™

BMI Calculation (ADULT)	BMI Percentile (AGES 2–20)	Ranking
BMI of 19 or under	Percentile of under 10 on chart	This is considered **underweight**. You should NOT be dieting or thinking about starting a diet plan!
BMI of 20 to 25	Percentile of 10 to 85 on chart.	This is the **healthy** range.
	Percentile of 85 to 95 on chart.	This range is considered **at risk** for becoming overweight. If you fall in this range, you're risking obesity and disease later in life.
BMI of 25 to 29.9	Percentile of greater than 95 on chart.	This is considered **overweight**. You're at great risk of obesity and disease later in life. Please check with your doctor about a safe, effective weight-loss program.
BMI of over 30	There is no "obese" category for youth.	This is considered **obese**. You're at great risk for lifelong obesity and re-lated illnesses. Please see your physician now to alter dietary habits, increase activity, and lose, then control, weight.

$$[165 \div (66 \times 66)] \times 703 = BMI$$
$$[165 \div 4356] \times 703 = BMI$$
$$.038 \times 703 = 26.714 \text{ (Your BMI is between 26 and 27.)}$$

Once you've calculated your BMI, compare that number against the BODY MASS INDEX-FOR-AGE graphs for boys and girls to twenty. These graphs, also developed by the NCHS in collaboration with the CDC, will show you how you compare to teens your age and gender. Once you've determined your percentile, use the chart below to see if you are underweight, overweight, or healthy. Most teens will fall within the healthy range.

The results of our sample calculation yielded a BMI between 26 and 27. This result falls in the "Overweight" category. However, BMI does not take into account the amount of muscle mass a person has, so it is not always accurate.

As you can see, there's a great diversity of heights and weights in teens—and all of them are completely normal! There are also varying body types and shapes, all just as normal.

Body Type

Maggie and Sharon are both five-foot-three, weigh 110 pounds, and wear size five.

"Pleeeeeease let me borrow your dress for the Christmas dance," Sharon pleads. "I promise I won't get anything on it!"

Maggie gives in, and Sharon borrows the red, strapless number Maggie wore to her cousin's wedding. One problem: when Sharon puts the dress on, it's too loose in the bust and too tight in the hips. It's a size five, though. So what's the problem?

Two words: body type. Body typing is defined not by how tall you are or how much you weigh, but how weight is distributed over your frame.

Chances are you've heard and used terms like short, chubby, tall, skinny, long-waisted, short-waisted, stacked, ripped, and even "skin and bones" to describe body types. Most of us do, but researchers, philosophers, and medical experts have developed other ways of describing the general shapes and sizes in which people come. These are called body types or **somatotypes**.

Different schools of thought exist on body typing. Depending on the philosophy, you can sort the human body into as few as three primary types and as many as twenty-five. Most of the systems that offer more classifications are linked to specific metaphysical, spiritual, or philosophical beliefs (for example, Ayurveda, a holistic school of medicine based on the ancient Vedic culture in India). Some, too, include categories that combine main classifications. For our purposes, we'll leave all those behind and examine the four basic somatotypes most medical doctors recognize: *android* (or mesomorph), *thyroid* (or ectomorph), *gynaeoid*, and *lymphatic* (or endomorph).

Each of these four body types—established by our genes—exhibit unique **metabolic** and hormonal characteristics. These characteristics define how our body stretches and fills out. Some body types easily store fatty deposits that dimple the skin (called **cellulite**). Other types build muscle easily. Some are predisposed to weight gain; a few fight against it. Still others tend to be lanky, bony, and resistant to bulky muscles.

Rarely is anyone distinctly one somatotype. Most people are a blend of two: a primary type tempered by traits

25

Sizing Up the Stars

Can you assign the correct body-type to each celebrity?

Sylvester Stallone
Robin Williams
Marilyn Monroe
Jimmy Stewart
Demi Moore
Oprah Winfrey
Courtney Cox
Jennifer Lopez

(Answers, top to bottom: android, lymphatic, gynaeoid, thyroid, android, lymphatic, thryoid, gynaeoid)

---

of a secondary. (Pure androids, thyroids, gynaeoids, and lymphatics are highly unusual and in the definite minority.)

Why is knowing your body type useful? It helps destroy myths and half-truths regarding what it means to be healthy, normal, and attractive. The fact is that we are all different shapes and sizes. No type is "perfect."

This knowledge is also important to maintaining ideal health. Whether you're an android, thyroid, gynaeoid, or lymphatic, you can impact your height-to-weight ratio, muscle density, and percentage of body fat through diet and exercise. (You cannot change bone structure, where fat is stored, or any tendency toward muscle bulk.) We need to focus on what is "healthy" for our particular body type, and not try to force ourselves to fit another type of body we can never achieve.

Lifestyle choices also impact the four body types. All four types can be underweight, overweight, "in shape," or "out of shape." For one or two body types, fitness is harder to maintain. That doesn't seem fair, but please keep in mind that despite what the media tells us, "pencil thin" is not always healthy. For example, men and women who *appear* to be thyroids, but who are really stockier androids—and have achieved their look through starvation—are *not* healthy. They're frequently gaunt,

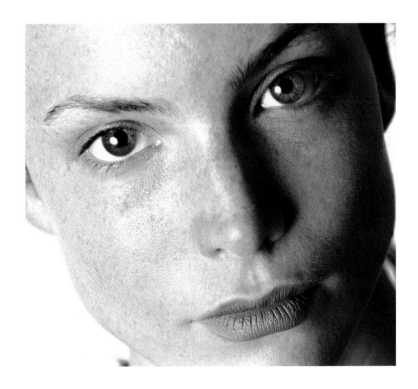

Celebrate the one and only you!

malnourished, even sick, and usually have problems with low energy, ***anemia***, and fatigue.

The One and Only You!

The next time you're tempted to compare your body (shape, weight, or height) to someone else's, know that your body is made to be uniquely yours. It has a predetermined height, a natural weight range, and a predestined rate at which it needs to mature. It's yours and yours alone. So far it's probably been pretty good to you, so try to learn to love and accept it. Here are some tips:

- Remember: despite Hollywood and fashion runways, *there's no such thing as the perfect figure . . . the perfect height . . . the perfect weight.* A daisy doesn't have to be a rose, nor a rose become a violet, to be beautiful. We're all different! The important thing is that we

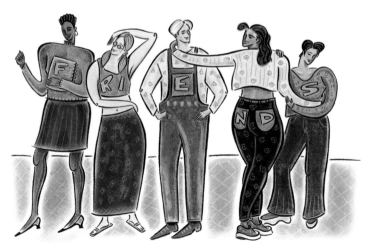

each strive to keep our unique body type in optimal condition *for that type*. Most of the time a healthy diet combined with regular exercise will achieve just that.

- Try embracing your less desirable traits. Don't just tolerate them; learn to love them! Every human body has pros and cons, strengths and weaknesses. It's the combination that makes you *you*!

- Set aside unrealistic expectations. We're all built differently, yet almost every boy or girl has at one time or another tried to fit into some twisted notion of what he or she "should" look like. It's unhealthy, not to mention futile, to alter what genetic heritage imposes. To be the best you, work only on that which you can change, and surrender to that which you can't.

Moving On

We've looked at general, physical growth shared by young men and women, and how varied it can be. Puberty—the process of becoming physically mature males and females—is equally varied, and this can affect height and weight. Some of the **pubertal** process is common to both sexes. Some is unique to each gender. We'll tackle shared changes first in chapter 3, then male and female development separately in chapter 4.

But before we move onto sexual maturity, we need to examine two additional and less obvious aspects of growth: intellectual and emotional development.

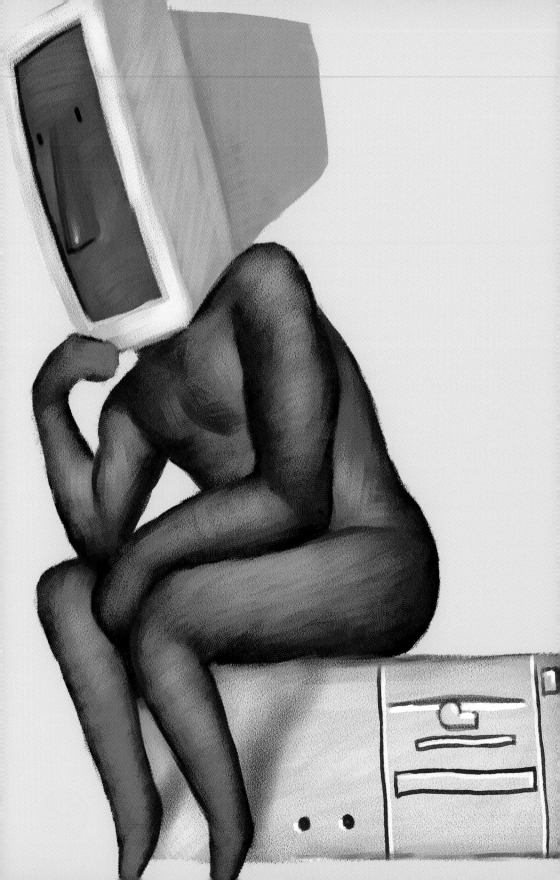

2
EXTREME MINDS:
Intellectual and Emotional Development

I *can't trust how I feel*, Jenny laments. *I've gotta be due for my period.*

Sometimes Jenny's irritable for no good reason. Other times she suddenly feels sad, then irrationally giggly. Plus, it seems as though all she does anymore is fight with her family. She wonders, *Why am I so angry all the time?* She used to enjoy hanging out with her parents, but now she can't stand to be seen with them. *They're sooooo embarrassing*, she finds herself thinking.

Do you ever feel like Jenny, embarrassed by your parents, annoyed by the smallest things, or suddenly giggling without knowing why? Do you suddenly find yourself so angry you can scream—and the next minute do you want to cry? You're in good company. An emotional roller coaster is perhaps *the* common rite of adolescence, regardless of size and shape.

As noted in the last chapter, teens change in more ways and more quickly than any other age group. These many, rapid, physical changes, combined with maturing

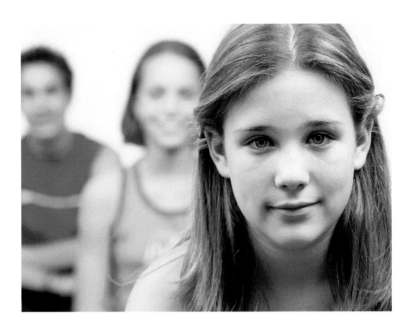

thought processes and raging hormones, often lead to emotional chaos. The mind is evolving rapidly during these years—**cognitively** and **psychosocially**—and this affects your emotions.

Cognitive Development

Simply said, cognitive development is how we think or the manner with which we process information and experiences.

According to the American Academy of Pediatrics, young children think concretely, that is, solely by what they know from direct experience. Abstract thinking is impossible. They can't generalize using one fact or combine ideas to form conclusions. Their perceptions are singular and immediate.

As children turn into adolescents (usually beginning by ages ten or twelve) they begin to think more like adults, applying logic and **relativity**. Abstract thought appears. Teens learn to form **hypotheses**, analyze contradicting facts, and approach problems systematically. **Causal relationships** begin to make sense to them, and anticipating **intangible** outcomes is added to their **repertoire** of thought. Adolescents begin to contemplate time spans like eternity and "deeper" concepts like purpose, worth, and death.

The moral code by which a teen will ultimately live also begins to take hold in adolescence. As his or her methods of thinking mature, discussions about religion, political ideas, and social issues emerge. Schoolwork becomes more complex. Concrete math tasks progress to abstract concepts like algebra and geometry. But not everyone develops at the same rate, and some adolescents may not be cognitively ready for these tasks. The pressure can be enormous. . . .

Jenny slams down the phone and rushes up the steps. She just found out that her best friend was selected for the advanced math track and she wasn't. Rita was always smarter, even more mature somehow, but now that they've hit middle school, that gap is widening. *Why can't I be more like Rita? I'm so stupid.*

Some teens develop thinking skills more quickly than others. (Remember our discussion of genes?) But most begin the journey to adult cognition by eleven or twelve. Over subsequent years, teens continue to hone adult-thinking behaviors, the bulk of which are in place by fifteen or sixteen years of age. For some, however, mental development will continue into young adulthood.

Physical development and cognitive development may or may not be on the same timetable. Such **synchrony** or **asynchrony** depends on genetic codes. The results of asynchrony (staggered developmental timetables) can be teens with child-like bodies and cognitively mature minds, or visa versa.

Lamar is physically mature for his fourteen years. So, too, is his thirteen-year-old girlfriend Louisa. Most of the kids at school think they're having sex.

"So have you 'done it'?" his friends ask.

"Sure," Lamar lies, hoping for admiration. He can't deny the sensations he feels when he's next to Louisa, but his head just can't take that step. These days, his mind and body are constantly at odds, and he's more uncertain of himself than ever. *I can't tell them I've never gone to first base, let alone home,* he silently groans.

34

They'll think I'm a loser . . . but what about Louisa? I really like her. With a twinge of conscience, Lamar continues, "Well, sort of."

The greatest problems occur when a teen is trapped in an adult body with a child's mind. This situation can lead to considerable inner conflict. For example: when the adult body wants to act on impulses to have unprotected sex, but the child mind can't grasp potential, long-term consequences like unwanted pregnancies or lifelong, sexually transmitted diseases (STDs). Or when the adult body wants to prove its virility by drinking hard or driving fast, but the child mind can't grasp issues like alcohol poisoning, injury, or even death. The results can be tragic.

Psychosocial Development

During cognitive development, most teens also begin to grow psychosocially. (Psychosocial development depends upon certain cognitive abilities being in place.) "Psychosocial" simply refers to a human's ability to relate healthfully to others and to the self. Pediatricians and psychiatrists agree that such abilities cover four general arenas:

1. Learning to effectively function independently of parents or caregivers (intellectually and emotionally).
2. Growing in self-awareness and developing an accurate self-image (including strengths and weaknesses).
3. Becoming capable of *mature* partnership in

35

    intimate relationships (responsible, honest, selfless, and respectful). *(This accomplishment isn't about the mere physical ability to have sex!)*

4. Possessing insight to set realistic life or career goals based on accurate self-image.

Because of its complexity, psychosocial development usually emerges over three distinct adolescent stages: early adolescence (ages 10 to 13), middle adolescence (ages 14 to 17), and late adolescence (ages 18 to 22). The age ranges indicated are not inflexible, but medical experts recognize them as reliable guides.

Individuation

The first two areas of psychosocial development—self-awareness and *individuation*, or separation from your parents—go hand-in-hand. Individuation depends on learning to see oneself accurately. Because forming self-image requires abstract thinking, and abstract thinking is part of cognitive development, cognitive ability must be in place—or at least evolving—for effective psychosocial development to occur.

    Most adolescents begin psychosocial growth by distancing from their caregivers. What this process looks like depends on the stage in which the teen is.

- In early adolescence (10–13), kids frequently exhibit distancing in irrational ways, mostly because necessary cognitive development isn't there yet. Tantrums (yes, like two-year-

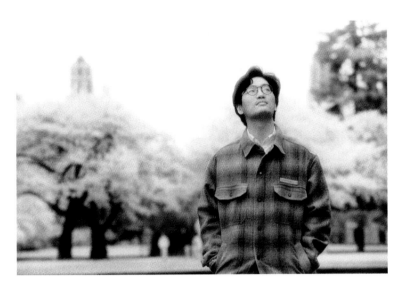

Growing up means learning how to be your own person.

olds!) are common, as is becoming inexplica-
bly clingy. One indicator that cognitive abilities are keeping up with psychosocial needs
is the young teen's embarrassment of his parents. That's a good sign! It means that the
child is starting to define himself as an individual, instead of as an extension of Mom or
Dad.

- In middle adolescence (14–17), teens tend to
  "distance" by starting to question or even
  challenge long-held, parent-taught beliefs
  about religion, politics, family structure, and
  love. Teens this age hunger to establish their
  own identities, and do so by individualizing
  their opinions, ideas, and beliefs. Varying degrees of rebellion are common.
- In late adolescence (18–22), young people

37

Break the Silence:
Ten Tips for Talking with Parents

1. Volunteer daily information, no matter how mundane, both good and bad. Don't make your parents ask.
2. Try shifting the focus back to them once in a while. Ask about their day!
3. Keep talking, no matter what. Try to talk about everyday stuff as often as you can to keep the line of communication open. (You might need it.)
4. If it's important, pick a good time to talk—for both of you—and plan what to say ahead of time. (The car is a great place!)
5. Be respectful in tone and word. Avoid sarcasm and "all or nothing" phrases like "You never . . ." or "You always. . . ."
6. Use "I" statements to communicate how you feel. (For example, instead of "You always cut me off!" try, "I feel like you're not really listening to me."
7. Avoid insulting your parents' opinions and beliefs. (For example, instead of "That's stupid!" try, "I don't agree and here's why.")
8. Don't make it personal. Words and ideas frustrate us, not people.
9. Don't take it personally. Your parents may be annoyed by a particular behavior of yours—but that doesn't mean they don't love you!
10. Accept them for who they are.

begin to understand that parents are simply people, that they're neither infallible and all-knowing nor all-powerful. One of the most interesting revelations at this age is that parents are suddenly less like parents and more like peers. The distancing is complete.

With increased ability to accurately interpret their world (cognitive development) and how they fit into it (psychosocial development), teenagers understandably long to explore who they are and branch out on their own. Independence, however, often feels insecure, lonely, and even a bit scary. That's perfectly normal.

Gradual independence provides the baby steps necessary to feel confident and capable. The key word here is "gradual." As frustrating as it is, parents must release the leash slowly for their children's physical safety and emotional well-being. They'd be negligent if they didn't.

Kevin is just dying to drive his friends to the game. "Mom, can I have your car next weekend to go to the game with Nick and Eddie?"

"Sure. Who's playing?"

"The Giants and the Eagles."

"Wait a minute. You mean a *pro* game? In the *city*?" his mom demands. "I thought you meant your high school game."

"Yeah. So what?" Kevin protests. "What's the difference?"

"The difference is three sixteen-year-old boys driving on a dangerously congested expressway, then tailgating with who knows who. No. You may not have my car."

Seething with frustration, Kevin explodes. "That's not fair! Eddie's parents let him drive *any*where!" He slams

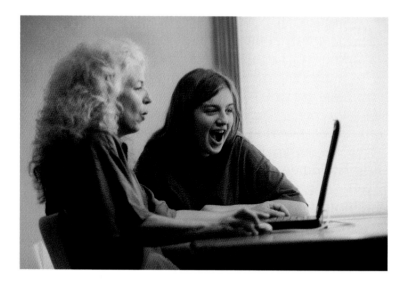

Relationships between parents and adolescents can be frustrating—but they can also be rewarding.

the door on his way out. "When are you gonna let me grow up?"

Living with parents can be frustrating. But think about it. Would you entrust a one-year-old nephew with that twenty in your wallet? Of course not! Why not? Because it would immediately go into his mouth. Not only could you lose your money, he could also choke on it and die.

What if he screams, cries, or shouts, "Not fair?" *He* thinks he's ready. Yet developmentally you know without a doubt that that toddler is simply not ready to handle cash, especially yours! For his sake and yours, you can't give in.

Down the Road:
Ten Tips for Shaping Your Future

1. Get to know yourself well. (What are your strengths? Weaknesses? Interests? Likes? Dislikes?) Be honest!
2. Take a skill or interest inventory, or read a book on the subject. (*What Color Is Your Parachute?* by Richard Nelson Bolles is one example.)
3. Divide a sheet of paper into two columns: one for your assets, strengths, and things you enjoy; the second for any disadvantages, weaknesses, and things you find draining. List each accordingly. Consider ideas that feed into the first column; discard ideas that would compound the second. Use what you learn to direct your planning for the future.
4. Talk to people you trust. Others can often see things in us that we can't. They can help identify strengths and weaknesses, and even steer you in directions you might otherwise have overlooked.
5. Be willing to explore multiple options. Be creative! Don't stop at the obvious; push your imagination!
6. Post your goal(s) where you'll see it (or them) every day. (This will keep you on track.)
7. Tackle only that which you can impact. Let go of the rest.
8. Ask questions. Explore financial, relational, and technological resources. Tap those resources!
8. Cultivate an optimistic attitude and tend to your self-esteem.
9. Don't take yourself too seriously!

Most teens sometimes behave like toddlers. They often want to take on a responsibility that, if they're honest, they're really not ready to handle physically, intellectually, or emotionally (that is, developmentally). "That's not fair!" is often the first phrase off their lips when they're denied an opportunity, and some teens just go ahead and do it anyway. Then the consequences of misinformed pride come back to haunt them in embarrassing moments, emotional hurts, mistakes, accidents, and even physical injury or death.

There's wisdom in taking things gradually! The first time you're home alone . . . the first time you meet friends at the mall without your parents . . . that first solo drive . . . your first date . . . your first weekend away at college. With each successful step into independence, you start shaping a more realistic, accurate, and positive self-image. You really are able to be your own person, separate from your parents!

As confidence grows in each stage of development, so do the ***incremental*** steps of leaving the nest. Gradual individuation is vital to healthy psychosocial development. For all concerned, it must be incremental.

Now consider what could have happened if your parents left you home alone at three, or let you go to the mall by yourself at seven, or gave you the car keys at ten. Too little too soon is deflating; too much too soon is defeating and can harm.

Progressing into independence doesn't have to mean World War III or damaged family relationships. If handled well, the process of distancing should ultimately, by the end of late adolescence, result in strong family ties based on mutual respect.

Self-Awareness

During younger years, notions of whom you would marry and who you'd become were based upon wistful thoughts or fantasies. By late adolescence, older teens are generally capable of forming realistic vocational, ed-

---

Ten Tips for Building Self-Esteem

1. Chuck the perfectionist! NO ONE is perfect. (Are your expectations too high?)
2. Journal. Write down at least one thing that pleases you about yourself for each trait that troubles you. (Everyone possesses something admirable.)
3. Acknowledge strengths to yourself and build on them. (Be honest!) You can!
4. If you can't change it (for example, your height), forget it! Don't waste another minute on it.
5. Replace each self-critical thought with an affirming one.
6. Don't overlook or minimize the inner beauty inside you and others. Outward appearances are temporary at best!
7. Take pride in your opinions and ideas, and voice them.
8. Help someone. Feeling like you're making a difference can work wonders.
9. Have fun! Make time for the people you care about and do the things you love.
10. Exercise! You'll reduce stress and be happier.

Shattering the Shell:
Seven Tips for Overcoming Shyness

1. Recognize you're not alone. Every teen experiences shyness sometime.
2. Lose the internal critic.
3. Focus on what you *can* offer. (What do you like about yourself?)
4. Learn social skills like eye contact, body language, asking questions, smiling, etc., one step at a time.
5. FAKE IT! Act as if you're not shy.
6. Plan ahead. Think about what to say or do in advance. (When it's time to face what you've been avoiding, you'll feel more self-confident.)

Remember: You're fine the way you are!

ucational, and lifestyle goals. The key is applying accurate self-understanding to long-term desires. Since some cognitive maturity is necessary for developing a realistic self-image, this area of psychosocial growth cannot evolve until cognitive skills and individuation are well established.

During early and mid-adolescence, your sense of self takes form. Genetics, family, friends, personal introspection, and the world are, by this point, shaping the adult "you." You know yourself pretty well now: strengths and weaknesses, relational tendencies and communication styles, loves and hates, plus needs and desires. You've also come to know your body and your mind.

A healthy self-esteem is based upon this knowledge. Self-esteem is the value with which a person views his or her qualities, character, abilities, and accomplishments.

The formation of effective aspirations considers all these things, too, and goal setting is merely one way to accomplish them. The trick is working with what you've been given. Remember, your view of yourself can and will affect goal setting and ultimately long-term results.

Everyone struggles with self-esteem sometimes, though, so knowing what destroys or builds it becomes important. Knowing you can build self-esteem (and how) is critical.

Pulling the Plug:
Nine Ways to Cool a Hot Head

1. Stop. Calm yourself. Think (*before* you say or do anything more).
2. Leave. Send yourself to your room. Take a time out.
3. Listen to music or soak in a bath (anything that's soothing).
4. Distract yourself. (Read. Do a craft. Watch a movie. Just don't stew.)
5. Write it down.
6. Work out. Exercise. (A good run does wonders.)
7. Punch pillows or shred tissues.
8. Meditate or practice deep breathing.
9. TALK ABOUT IT (with someone you trust). Try to be rational.

COMMON EMOTIONS

A most rewarding experience of adolescence is one day realizing you're an independent, responsible young adult. But getting there is tough. Your body is transforming in countless ways, your thought processes are changing, and your social abilities are maturing. Even your most private feelings seem to be taking on lives of their own. No wonder you're an emotional heap sometimes!

Jon has been thinking about the new girl all month. When he finally spots her in the cafeteria, he takes a deep breath, hopes he doesn't smell, and heads her way. As he approaches, two perfect brown eyes meet his, and suddenly he can't breathe. *What am I going to say? What if she thinks I'm a jerk?* Gathering his courage, he keeps walking . . . right past her to the display cabinet along a nearby wall. He feigns interest in the gold faces staring back at him from atop the trophies. Mentally, he scolds himself, *You're such a wimp!*

Shyness is a social emotion that impacts the whole person. It affects thoughts, words, and deeds. It is fueled by feelings of awkwardness, discomfort, self-consciousness, insecurity, nervousness, and even fear. You might not think of yourself as shy, but if you find yourself hesitating to say or do something because of what others might think, shyness is most likely to blame.

Even though there are personality types that lend themselves to shyness, almost every teen goes through times of being shy. The good news is that no one is condemned for life! Shyness waxes and wanes throughout adolescence. If you're in a shy time, try surrounding yourself with supportive people. Knowing someone is behind you can help.

46

Five Common Mood Swings in Every Teen

1. shy and tentative to outgoing and friendly
2. irritable and angry to lighthearted and giddy
3. blue or depressed to cheerful or optimistic
4. insecure or anxious to confident and indifferent
5. stressed and overwhelmed to carefree and calm

A second, universal, adolescent emotion is anger. Why do so many teens fly off the handle so quickly? Often stress, powerlessness, or insecurity is the culprit. Other causes could be hormones, lack of sleep, or even personality. Whatever the cause, you *will* get angry. Everyone does, so we need to learn how to deal with it.

Please remember that there's nothing wrong with feeling mad. In fact, anger can be healthy, particularly when it's masking primary feelings like jealousy, hurt, or frustration. It's how you handle your anger that makes the difference.

Other common emotions include anxiety, fear, the blues, depression, insecurity, embarrassment, competitiveness, joy, elation, excitement, love, hate, and loneliness. You can experience any or all of these in just one day! (For further information, please see *Surviving the Roller Coaster: A Teen's Guide to Coping with Moods*, another book in this series.)

Such drastic mood swings are normal for teens. One of the primary culprits is puberty. Chapter 3 will tell you more.

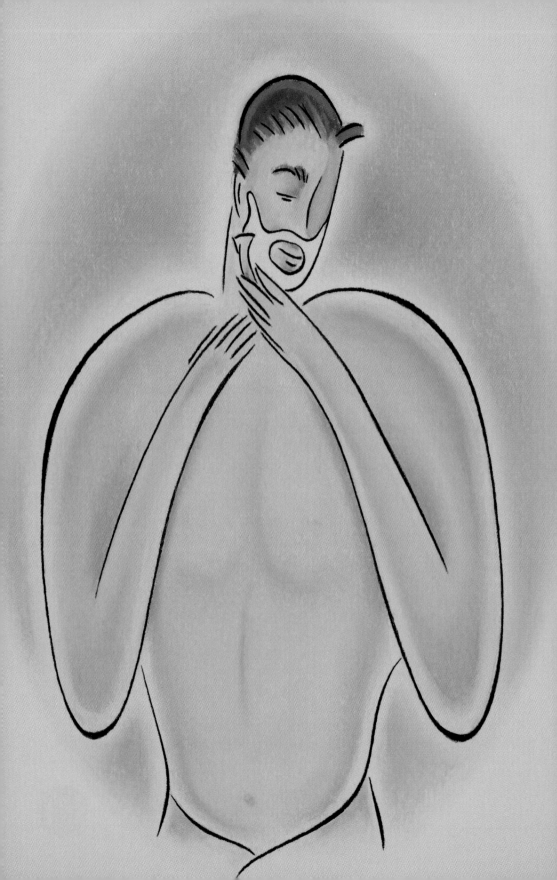

3
EXTREME CHANGES:
General Pubertal Development

Puberty is the stage of development in which a young person sexually matures, becoming capable of reproduction. We've been discussing adolescence, and technically puberty is part of adolescence, the sexual maturation part. Whereas adolescence covers the whole package, however, including both body and mind, puberty deals with just the body. And because adolescence includes cognitive and psychosocial development, it usually lasts much longer than puberty itself, hence the asynchrony discussed in the last chapter. Puberty generally takes about four years to complete.

Whether you're a guy or girl, puberty is a time of dramatic changes in your body. These changes affect height, weight, and body mass, as discussed in chapter 1, but puberty produces other changes as well. You might notice hair growing in new places, breast development (guys, too!), strange odors and even a change in your complexion. Some developments will be unique to girls, and others to guys. (We discuss each separately in the next chapter.) This chapter focuses on changes common to both.

Let's start with what triggers the onset of puberty. At just the right time for you, your brain releases higher levels of a hormone that signals the rest of your body to start puberty. It acts like a green light or starter pistol. This hormone is called gonadotropin-releasing hormone (GnRH for short). When GnRH reaches your ***pituitary gland***, it tells this gland to release two more pubertal hormones: luteinizing hormone (LH for short) and follicle-stimulating hormone (FSH for short). Males and females both have both hormones. Your gender determines the way in which they each go to work on your body. (See chapter 4.)

For girls, puberty can commence as early as age seven and as late as age thirteen, but most girls begin the journey around age ten. (African American girls tend to start a year or so earlier than other girls.) In general, puberty in girls lasts four years, but can stretch out to six or more years or be done in just two. Most young women complete puberty, or are sexually mature, by fifteen years of age.

At fifteen, Amanda is gorgeous. With an hourglass figure, clear complexion, full lips, and silken black hair, she gets more attention from others than she'd like. Her twin brother isn't as lucky. He still looks much like he did at twelve, except disproportionately taller, with large feet and hands. His shoulders haven't widened; he has yet to shave; and his face occasionally breaks out. These two are twins. So what's going on?

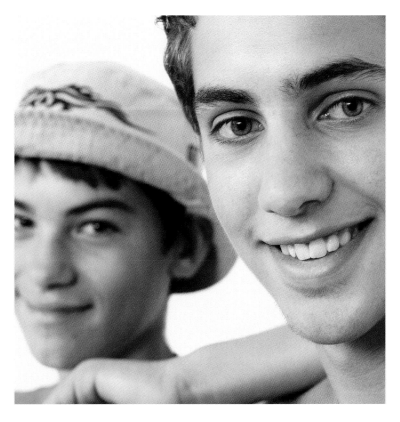

Right On Schedule

Boys tend to lag behind girls by one to two years, starting puberty as early as nine and as late as fourteen, but most begin by around eleven or twelve. For guys the process averages three years, but can range from two to five years. Most young men will complete puberty, or be sexually mature, by age sixteen.

Most adolescents enter puberty according to these guidelines, but a few experience **precocious** puberty (early puberty) or delayed puberty (late puberty). In most cases, either variation is just an extension of normal puberty. Sometimes, though, a medical reason can be responsible. (For example, malnutrition can cause delayed puberty.) Early and late puberty tend to be genetic, or run in families.

"Look. There's David Gunning!" Linda points her finger.

It's the first day of ninth grade after a long summer break. "What a hunk!" Linda says. "He must have grown a whole foot over summer vacation!"

"Is that really David?" Susan asks. "Wow. He looks really different!"

Puberty does affect height. In fact, it is during puberty that most teens, particularly boys, experience their greatest growth spurts. Boys can expect to grow nearly ten inches over these years, or up to three or five inches per year! Girls usually experience their greatest growth spurt one or two years into puberty, immediately before they start menstruating. They top out at two to four inches per year. Most girls grow only two or three additional inches once menstruation begins.

During puberty, the majority of teens ultimately tally seven to ten inches (23–28 cm) of growth before reaching full adult height. Some can grow slightly more even after puberty is complete. Growth only stops when the bones' growth plates fuse in the latter half of adolescence. Be-

Bones and Backpacks

Your leg and arm bones are not the only bones growing as you get taller. So are your vertebrae. How can you make life easier on that developing spine? Here are five "health" tips for selecting and using the ever-popular backpack:

1. Choose a pack with two, wide, well-padded shoulder straps and hip belt.
2. Start a trend: USE the hip belt. It distributes weight so that hips and legs bear more of the load.
3. Resist slinging your backpack over one shoulder. Use both shoulder straps.
4. Bend your knees when hoisting it to your shoulders.
5. Limit the load to no more than ten percent of your body weight.
6. Consider a backpack on wheels.

sides the obvious changes these years bring about—height, weight, and sexual development—there are a number of less noticeable changes that occur. Here are a few.

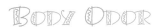

Body Odor

Have you noticed that you sweat more now than when you were a kid, even when it's not hot? Maybe you've

53

Foul Feet

Foot odor can be *really* embarrassing. If you have smelly feet, you're not alone. Lots of people do. Try these steps for offing odors:

- Wash feet daily, even between your toes.
- Apply a combination deodorant/antiperspirant to your feet.
- Dust feet with baking soda before putting on clean, absorbent socks.
- Choose well-ventilated shoes. (Nylon sneaks breathe better than leather.)
- Change socks with each wear and allow shoes to air out completely before wearing them again.
- If all else fails, try odor-absorbing shoe inserts.
- See your medical practitioner if problem persists. (You may have athlete's foot.)

even become aware of strange, new smells wafting from different areas of your body. That's body odor. Contrary to popular belief, this odor is produced not from sweat itself, but when sweat reacts to bacteria on the skin.

You've always had sweat glands, even as a small child. During puberty, though, they become more active. Sweat glands are all over your body, but concentrated in the armpits, feet, and groin. (Isn't that what usually smells?) As unsettling as they can be, these odors are easily dealt with.

The best way to control body odor is to take a bath or shower daily. Washing removes any bacteria and dirt that collect on your skin. Remember: if there's no bacteria with which to react, there's no odor!

You should also change underwear and socks every day. Since the feet and groin area are sweat-gland centers, changing this apparel is a must. Also, natural fibers like cotton tend to keep you drier than synthetics like nylon or polyester. To prevent odor—and even urinary or vaginal infections—all underpants (even thongs) should have at least a cotton crotch.

Armpit sweat tends to react more strongly with skin bacteria than other types of sweat your body produces; hence its stronger odor. Almost everyone has underarm odor, and it's usually easily managed. T-shirts, like underpants, should be cotton and changed daily, but the use of deodorant and antiperspirant is largely cultural. Most Americans use one or the other. Antiperspirants reduce or stop sweating, but not odor. Deodorants cover the odor, but will not prevent sweating. Many products combine the two.

The Skin Scoop

- Skin is our largest organ.
- Skin functions as a barrier, keeping harmful substances and microorganisms (like bacteria) out and vital body fluids in.
- Eyelids have the thinnest skin.
- The soles of our feet have the thickest.
- Skin on an average, 150-pound adult weighs in at about nine pounds.
- That same skin, if stretched flat, would cover approximately two square yards.
- Americans spend $260 million per year on over-the-counter (OTC) skin-care medications.

55

Pimple Prevarications

1. Outbreaks are caused by diet. WRONG! Studies have not found a single connection between diet and acne.
2. Stress causes pimples. WRONG! Day-to-day stress has nothing to do with it.
3. Acne is contagious. WRONG! Nothing you do can either cause you to develop acne nor give it to someone else.
4. Pimples are caused by poor hygiene. WRONG! Skin cells lining hair follicles shed constantly and usually travel harmlessly to the skin's surface where they're washed away. When they mix with oil and bacteria in the pores, they can form a plug and never get there. That mix, not dirt, causes a pimple.
5. Tanning helps. WRONG! In fact, the sun can dry and irritate skin, leading to future breakouts.

SKIN

The increase of pubertal hormones running through your body not only triggers sexual development, but also causes your skin to produce more oil. You might notice oily patches of skin, particularly on your face, which you've never noticed before. You may start getting pimples. When oil glands are more active, pores can clog with the extra oil, causing whiteheads and blackheads. When the pore gets infected, that's when you get a pimple.

Aggravating Acne: Five Factors in Flare-ups

- Fluctuating hormone levels in both guys and girls
- Premenstrual changes to hormone levels
- Environmental irritants like pollution and humidity
- Vigorous scrubbing
- Frequently touching skin

Almost no one makes it through adolescence without getting pimples. Many teens develop at least some degree of acne. The National Institute of Health (NIH) estimates nearly 85 percent of young people ages twelve

Alleviating Acne: Five Tips for Preventing Breakouts

1. Wash pillowcases, sheets and blankets often. Washing gets rid of dead skin cells and oils that build up on the fabric as you sleep.
2. Remove make-up before sleeping. Pay attention to hard-to-reach places like around the nostrils.
3. When buying make-up, choose brands that say noncomedogenic or nonacnegenic on the label.
4. If you wear glasses or sunglasses, clean frames and the nose bridge often to prevent bacteria and oil residue from clogging pores around your eyes and nose.
5. Drink plenty of water, at least six glasses a day. It flushes out impurities.
6. Keep oily hair gels or spray off face.
7. Wash off sweat.

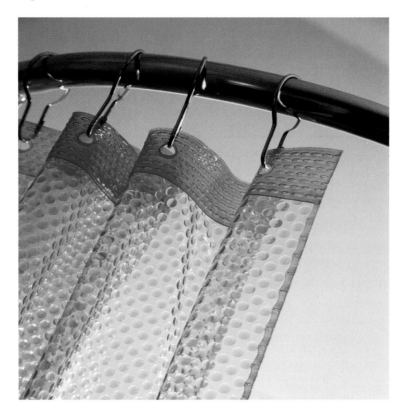

Showering every day is a good way to fight pimples.

through twenty-four develop some level of this skin condition. Most cases clear up by the late teens.

Pimples most frequently appear on the face, but they also commonly form on the neck, back, chest, and shoulders. Stray ones can occasionally appear on your arms, legs, or buttocks. No matter where they pop up, all pimples are infections.

The key to preventing pimples is reducing excess oil that accumulates on the skin. The less oil, the less chance of blocked pores! How? By washing prone areas twice a day with mild soap and warm water, then rinsing with clean, cool water. (Warm water widens the pores for deep cleaning, and cool water closes them again.) Try not to scrub too hard, because irritating your skin can trigger the release of even more oil, creating more pimples.

Even with the best skin care, everyone gets pimples sometime during puberty. As tempting as it is, don't pick or pop them! Squeezing or popping can inflame the infection. Check at your local pharmacy or grocery store. There are many effective, over-the-counter (OTC) ointments and cleansers that can help outbreaks clear up more quickly.

Myths abound about what causes pimples and what helps heal them. If you are worried about your complexion, see your doctor or a reputable **_dermatologist_**. They can prescribe stronger medications to manage your skin care. In the mean time, keep your face clean!

The Truth About Tresses

- The life cycle of head hair is broken into two stages: active growth and rest. Active growth can last several years, while the resting stage is sixty to ninety days.
- A normal scalp holds 100,000 hairs, with up to 15 percent in the resting stage.
- Once in resting mode, the hair sheds soon.
- Most heads average a hair-loss rate of seventy-five hairs per day.
- Hair grows more quickly in the daytime and summer.
- Hair grows more slowly at night and in winter.

Hair

Another subtle change of puberty can be found in your hair. In chapter 4, we'll discuss body hair, but here we're referring to the hair on your head. You might notice that it needs washing more frequently, or that once dry hair is now oily.

Pores on your scalp secrete the same oils as skin pores elsewhere on your body. Because pubertal hormones trigger the skin *every*where to produce more oil, your head's skin—your scalp—is also producing more oil. Every teen encounters this problem.

This oil keeps hair healthy and shiny when it's present in just the right amount. Too much oil, however, makes hair look greasy or dirty. Not enough, and the hair can become dry or brittle.

If your hair tends to be dry, try to limit yourself to shampooing only once or twice per week. Infrequent washing allows natural oils to build up and condition the hair. Make sure you use a moisturizing shampoo and conditioner. That should help.

If your hair tends to be oily, wash it every day, and use shampoos designed for oily hair. Also pay attention to labels. Some of your hair care products (mousse, gels, etc.) may be adding oils to your hair that you don't need.

Teeth and Breath

Ah . . . that first kiss: it sounds romantic, doesn't it? Now imagine kissing someone who doesn't brush his or her teeth. Thick, yellow ***plaque***. Food particles. Pasty, bad breath. Yuk.

As you made your way through childhood, your **deciduous** (or baby) teeth (all twenty of them) first came in, then fell out again one by one, as permanent teeth pushed up to take their place. By mid-puberty, age fourteen or older, you likely have twenty-eight of your permanent teeth in place. The last four, commonly known as wisdom teeth, usually erupt during late adolescence, when you're between seventeen and twenty-one years of age. Those four complete the set of thirty-two secondary (or permanent) teeth. And all thirty-two need care.

Some teeth come in straight, with room to spare. Some grow in crooked, rotated, or overlapping. If there's not enough space for the teeth to come in, wisdom teeth may not erupt at all, while others shift into crooked positions. Such misalignment is a concern for two reasons.

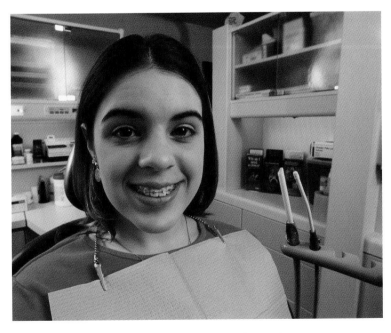

Braces are designed to correct tooth misalignments.

61

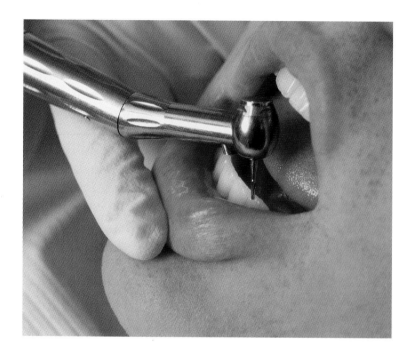

Regular visits to the hygienist minimize the build-up of plaque on your teeth.

The first is functional. Misaligned teeth can interfere with proper chewing. Plus, they're harder to brush well and keep clean. Bacteria-laden plaque builds up in the hard-to-reach places, leading to bad breath, greater tooth decay, or other dental problems down the road.

Another concern is more psychological. People with crooked teeth sometimes feel self-conscious about them. They may even hesitate to laugh or smile for fear of exposing their teeth. That's sad and unnecessary.

Most dentists can tell if a patient's adult teeth will be misaligned by the time he or she is six or seven years old. If they suspect any problem, they will usually refer the patient to an **orthodontist** for corrective treatment like braces. Any referral to an orthodontist, though, must wait until the patient is closer to his or her teen years when the permanent teeth are in place. Consequently, braces are a common sight in adolescence.

With or without braces, oral hygiene is critical. A healthy diet (light on acids and sugars) can make a big difference, but brushing, flossing, and regular check-ups are critical to caring for one's mouth.

The American Dental Association (ADA) recommends brushing for a minimum of two minutes at least twice a day (morning and bedtime), but preferably after every meal. You should also brush after eating anything high in sugar, or leave at least three-hour intervals between high sugar foods like soda. Flossing needs to be done once a day to remove plaque and particles that brushing can't get.

Because plaque is a translucent film of bacteria, and bacteria in the mouth is a main cause of bad breath, brushing and flossing well are perhaps the most effective means of maintaining fresh breath. Your entire mouth— not just teeth, but also gums, and tongue—should be brushed. That person you kiss will thank you.

Fatigue

If you've started puberty, chances are you're not getting enough sleep. There's a lot going on in your body right now, and it knows it.

All those changes are taxing and demand more sleep, so most teens' brains tell the internal sleep regulator—or **circadian** rhythm—to sleep later. The extra sleep allows

---

Are You Getting Enough Sleep?

Test yourself. How long does it take you to fall asleep? If it takes you fifteen minutes or more to doze off, you're probably getting enough. If you fall asleep in less than five or ten minutes (or during the day in the most embarrassing places!), you may be running on a sleep deficit.

---

for the release of more growth hormone. This hormone helps tissues grow properly and promotes bone growth.

Additionally, another rampant hormone—melatonin, one that triggers sleep—is produced (prompting sleep) at different times of the day for teens than for adults and children. Teens' bodies are actually *wired* to sleep differently! So the next time Mom or Dad has a hard time dragging you out of bed, blame your hormones.

Most teens are forced to fight their internal clocks because school, church, and work demand early rising. That seems so unfair! But it can help to know how much sleep a body really needs to stay healthy during this stage of development.

Most teens need about nine or nine and a half hours of sleep *every night* to stay healthy. Not surprisingly, many surveys show that 25 percent of average teens get only six to seven hours a night. Such chronic sleep deprivation can lead to difficulty waking, sleeping in class, inability to concentrate, falling grades, and even depression.

Fatigue from lack of sleep and strenuous physical activity is to be expected. Other causes are more emotional: stress, worry, anxiety, anger, love, excitement, and other intense emotions.

Why can't I sleep? Roger tosses and turns. He looks again at the clock. *I need to be up in just three hours. . . . I'm never going to be okay.* Tomorrow's the big game, plus a huge math test, but no matter how hard he tries, Roger just can't force himself to sleep.

Everyone has a night of insomnia sooner of later. This type of isolated and occasional type of sleeplessness is called transient insomnia. It is perfectly normal. If, though, sleeplessness occurs for a few weeks or longer, two or more nights per week, then you might have **chronic** insomnia and should see your doctor.

Those are the main areas in which both girls and boys will notice more subtle changes of puberty. In the next chapter, we'll tackle the primary change puberty brings:

Sleep Stats

- Twenty percent of high school students report falling asleep in class.
- Fifty percent of teens report being most alert after 3:00 p.m.
- Only 15 percent of American teens get eight hours or more sleep nightly.
- Drivers under twenty-five have the highest probability of sleep-related accidents.

---

sexual maturity. As you've probably already noticed, sexual development is quite different for boys and girls.

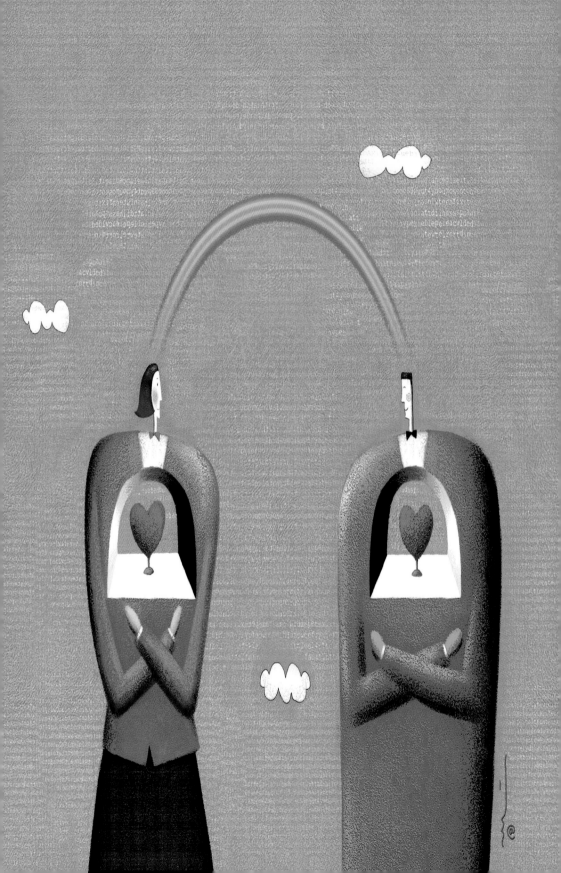

A Peek at Puberty

YOUNG WOMEN	YOUNG MEN
Breast buds appear.	Testes enlarge.
Pubic hair starts to grow.	Pubic hair starts to grow.
Vagina, labia, and clitoris enlarge.	Scrotum enlarges and darkens.
Body odor becomes noticeable.	Body odor becomes noticeable.
Underarm and leg hair grows.	Underarm and leg hair grows.
Growth spurt hits.	Growth spurt hits.
Acne sets in.	Acne sets in.
Hips widen.	Shoulders broaden and muscles grow larger.
Pubic hair thickens over pubic mound.	Pubic hair thickens over pubic mound.
Breasts fill out to adult size.	Penis and testes lengthen to adult size.
Menstruation begins.	Nocturnal emissions start to wane.
Ovulation becomes regular.	Testes produce sperm.
Height increases by 1" or 2".	Voice deepens.

Right On Schedule

That's the basics for both genders. The rest of this chapter is divided into two sections: one section on female sexual development, followed by a section on male sexual development. The two genders, as different as they are, follow surprisingly similar paths to maturity.

Extreme Girls: Becoming Women

What's that? Kelly wonders as she washes in the shower. Looking down, she sees a few stray hairs growing on her lower pelvis. Her nipples have also been a little tender lately. *Wow*, she thinks.

The changes Kelly is noticing can begin anytime between seven and thirteen years of age. (See chapter 3.) Such changes mark the early stages of puberty.

First Things First

Most girls initially notice breast buds: small, tender lumps beneath each nipple. This beginning stage of breast development signals the official start of puberty in girls, regardless of age. Nipples might be slightly tender and noticeable through shirts now, so this is the time some girls start wearing training bras.

Some girls might notice that one breast is larger than the other. This lopsidedness can cause concern, but it needn't. Breast buds often appear first on one side, then

70

- Hair grows everywhere on the human body except on our eyelids, lips, palms of our hands, and soles of our feet.
- Eighty-one percent of American women remove underarm and leg hair.
- Only 51 percent of European women remove underarm and leg hair.
- Electrolysis and laser hair removal are options for permanently removing hair. Check first with your medical practitioner.

is also the time that underarm odor and foot odor develop.

One to Two Years Later . . .

Pubic hair is now fully established and breasts are slightly fuller. Perhaps the most exciting aspect of this stage (for many girls) is the growth spurt. A teenage girl's fastest growth, or peak height velocity, happens now. She can shoot up a few inches in just one year! Arms, legs, hands, and feet get bigger. Even her pelvis widens (in preparation for later childbirth).

Body fat also increases in this stage—distressing to many teen girls—distributing in greater proportion to the hips and breasts. Consequently, the mid-pubescent female takes on a more womanly shape, with rounded hips and fuller breasts. As her breasts fill out, her nipples and areola (the surrounding, circular, brown area) enlarge and get darker.

Please note that weight gain and reproportioning in this stage is healthy and expected. Any dieting to slow or stop the progression is foolish and could be dangerous. A womanly shape is attractive!

The culminating event of mid-puberty, usually after peak height velocity is reached, is the arrival of a young woman's first period, or menarche. Most girls begin menstruation about two and a half years after the first breast buds appear. However, periods, or cycles of menstrual bleeding, often remain somewhat unpredictable and irregular for up to eighteen months after they start. That's normal.

Remember the ovaries? (The organ that released estrogen to get puberty really on its way?) Well, girls are born with two ovaries. Each ovary holds thousands of eggs, or ova. Your ovaries don't "produce" eggs; they merely release them when the time is right. (You have all the eggs you're going to get when you're born.) These ova are there for the purpose of reproduction.

What do eggs have to do with menstruation? During one menstrual cycle, the uterus (also called the womb) begins building up its lining with extra blood and tissue, hoping to nourish a fertilized egg. About one to two weeks after this build up begins, an egg (ovum) is released from one ovary—ovaries usually alternate month to month—and travel down the fallopian tube to the waiting uterus.

If an egg reaches the uterus and is fertilized there by a man's sperm, it embeds in the uterine wall and a fetus grows. If the egg is not fertilized, then the uterus doesn't need the extra blood and tissue any longer. This unused build up tears away from the uterine wall and gets discharged through the vagina in what is called a period. A period usually lasts from five to seven days, but the entire menstrual cycle normally takes about twenty-eight.

74

Sanitary Sense

- Tampons are worn internally, inside the vagina. Pads (or sanitary napkins) are worn externally, attached to your underpants with a self-adhesive strip.
- Both are equally effective for absorbing blood.
- Both leak, although tampons are easier to keep in place.
- Both tampons and pads come in varying sizes to accommodate varying levels of blood flow (usually thin or light, regular, super, and maxi or ultra).
- Using a tampon does not affect virginity.
- Toxic shock syndrome (a bacterial infection) is not a risk with pads. It is a very slight risk with tampon use, particularly if tampons are not changed frequently.
- Both tampons and pads should be changed every four to six hours.

However, some women's cycles take only twenty-one days, and others need as long as forty-two days to complete. That's a wide range, all of which doctors consider normal.

The amount of blood lost with each period can vary widely. Sometimes you'll have a heavy flow and have to use more sanitary products than normal. Other times you'll have a light flow and use less. The heaviest flow usually takes place at the onset.

You've probably heard of PMS, or premenstrual syndrome. PMS is simply a fancy name for a collection of symptoms some women experience one or two weeks before the start of their periods. Hormonally driven, these symptoms can include irritability, moodiness, sadness, headaches, back pain, bloating, and breast tenderness. Most young women have some or all of these symptoms, while a few don't have any at all. Symptoms usually last up to a week preceding the period and disappear once the period starts. If this is a big problem for you, talk to your health care provider.

> *"Women complain about PMS, but I think of it as the only time of the month I can be myself."*
>
> —Roseanne Barr

When your periods have settled into a regular cycle, start to track them by marking the first day of bleeding on your calendar. If you count twenty-eight days from that day, you'll have a good idea when to expect your next period. Knowing when to expect it can help in packing for a weekend away or vacation. (Doctors also need this information at annual check-ups.) Ovulation (when the ovary releases an egg) generally happens fourteen to seventeen days from that first day. This is the time you're most fertile, or have the best chances of getting pregnant.

GOING . . . GOING . . . GONE!

You might think that puberty for a girl ends with her first period. Not so! It can take up to eighteen more months for ovulation to begin in earnest, even if there's a period. But as the reproduction system makes these final adjustments, other changes begin to wane and wrap up.

The majority of teen girls achieve full, adult breast size by the end of puberty, although breasts can grow and shape for about four years after a first period. Final breast size is determined by heredity (or genes) and can range from very small (bra cup size AA) to very full (EE). Nipples become more elevated atop the breasts, and the areola finishes expanding. Please note: women's breasts vary greatly, and all sizes and shapes are normal, including yours.

Breast tenderness and abdominal pain often accompany monthly periods now. Cramps are caused by the uterus contracting as it tries to shed its unused build up of blood and tissue. From here on out, you can expect

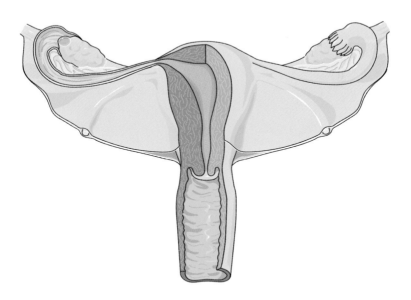

The ovaries, uterus, and vagina.

77

> ## Freaky Facts
>
> • No human features that come in pairs are exactly the same size. Not legs, arms, ears, eyes or even breasts and testes.
> • A protruding Adam's apple is unique to men. You'll never see one on a woman.
> • About 25 percent of adult women have breasts of noticeably different size.

regular periods—barring pregnancy—for the next thirty to forty years.

Most girls will only grow another one or two inches in height once menstruation begins. That's all. The growth spurt is over.

At this point, the older adolescent is considered sexually mature. That little girl is gone, replaced by a woman fully capable of reproducing, that is, conceiving and bearing a child. But remember, being physically able to have and enjoy sex doesn't mean that the mind is ready. Cognitive and psychosocial development are still plugging along, and may lag behind pubertal development by several years! (See chapter 2.)

Extreme Guys: Becoming Men

Kurt gazes at the stranger in the mirror. For the first time he's noticing that he looks older. A more angular face, slightly stubbled, returns his stare. *When did I change?* he wonders. *I don't feel any different . . .*

For some teens, puberty seems to take hold overnight. One day they're a little kid chasing kites. The next, they're dating. Boys are no exception.

First Things First

Whereas breast buds signaled the beginning of puberty in girls, testicular enlargement defines the start of puberty in young men. When *testicles* are more than one inch long, puberty has definitely begun. These testicles

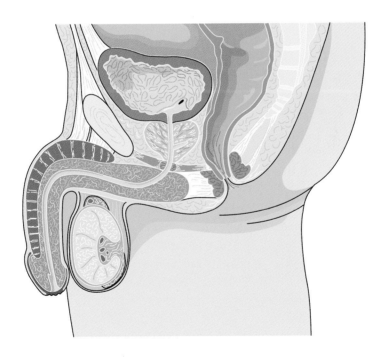

The male reproductive organs develop during puberty.

continue to grow throughout puberty, nearly doubling their length.

The testes' job is to produce sperm for procreation and testosterone for male development. Like women's breasts, they can be different sizes. The right testis is usually larger than the left, and the left usually sits lower in the **scrotum** than the right. Such asymmetry is perfectly normal.

In order to effectively produce sperm, the testes must be kept about six degrees cooler than internal body temperature (or about 92 degrees Fahrenheit and 34 degrees Centigrade). So, unlike women's ovaries, testicles cannot be internal. That's where the scrotum comes in.

The scrotal sac hangs outside the body, behind the penis. This sac holds the testes. Its main job is to protect each testis and regulate temperature by contracting and expanding in response to heat or cold. On cold days, the scrotum shrinks and tightens around the testes to retain heat. When hot, it becomes loose and floppy to vent excess heat. These responses happen involuntarily. You can't help it.

After the testicles begin to grow, the scrotum darkens and pubic hair appears. This hair, fine and sparse at first, usually begins to grow near the base of the penis. As with girls, it eventually spreads upward and outward in a triangular formation, gradually thickening and darkening as it goes. Ultimately, this hair becomes coarse and curly.

The penis also starts to grow about this time. Pre-pubertal penis length is about two inches, but boys can expect their penises to continue to grow over the next four years, more than doubling in size. Full penile length is not reached until the later stages of puberty.

Leg hair, underarm hair, and body odor also develop in early puberty. Facial hair is the last to come in. You probably don't need to worry about shaving yet, but now is the time to check out antiperspirants and deodorants. Your friends will thank you!

One last note: approximately 64 percent of early pubescent boys will notice some extra tissue or "lumps" around one or both nipples. The nipples might even become tender. This condition, called gynecomastia, is caused by breast tissue (yes, you have breast tissue) responding to pubertal hormones. It's quite common, normal, and no cause for concern. You're not developing female breasts! This physical reaction usually lasts less than a year and gradually goes away on its own.

One or Two Years Later

Like his female counterpart, a boy's growth accelerates in mid-puberty. At peak height velocity, boys can grow four or five inches per year! Shoulders also widen and become more muscular. Weight gain and redistribution is normal and should be expected. Again, dieting to prevent it is unhealthy and can result in delayed puberty and a decrease in height development.

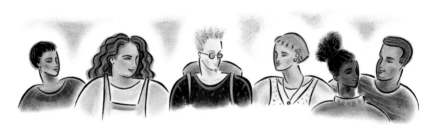

During this time, some boys become concerned over a perceived lack of muscular development. Take heart! Muscle growth continues long after peak height is reached, sometimes for years.

The testicles and penis continue to lengthen during this time. By now, the testes are efficiently producing sperm and will continue to do so for the rest of a man's life. Sperm is produced at a rate of hundreds of millions each day!

As the testes produce sperm, the sperm travels out of each testis, down a long, coiled tube called the epididymis (pronounced ep-uh-DID-uh-miss) where sperm develop, then out the scrotum via the vas deferens (pronounced vahs-DEF-uh-rinz). The vas deferens connects the epididymis to the urethra, the tube that carries semen and urine out of the penis. Millions of sperm travel through the vas deferens each day. Since sperm build up there, it's sometimes called the sperm storehouse.

Semen is the fluid that leaves a man's penis when he ejaculates. Unlike sperm, semen does not originate in the testes. Rather it is the product of combined fluids from the prostate gland (pronounced PRAH-state) and seminal vesicles. Upon ejaculation, sperm flood out of the vas deferens, mixing with semen in the urethra, and squirt out the tip of the penis. Each time a man ejaculates, up to 500 million sperm are released!

The alarm buzzes. Andrew stirs. Fumbling for the snooze button, he rolls over and notices a wet, sticky feeling in his pants. He knows it's not urine, but what is it?

Chances are Andrew has had a wet dream or nocturnal emission. Teen boys experience such emissions during puberty when their bodies start producing testosterone. Wet dreams occur during sleep, when a boy dreams about something sexual. Although some boys feel embarrassed (or even guilty) about wet dreams, they really shouldn't. Most guys experience nocturnal emissions at some point during puberty. Plus these emissions are completely involuntary. Boys can't help having them.

Some boys may have several erections during sleep. An erection is a lengthening and hardening of the penis that occurs as penile tissues fill up with blood. The penis actually stands up or becomes erect. For reproductive purposes, the penis must be hard and long to enter the vagina and deposit sperm.

What triggers an erection? Sometimes there's no apparent reason at all—even infants have erections—but many erections are caused by visual or *tactile* stimulation. Either way, erections can wane on their own or upon ejaculation, as with wet dreams. Wet dreams lessen over pubertal years, and eventually stop.

Another disconcerting change for mid-pubertal guys is hearing their voices crack. While talking, a boy might experience his voice fluctuate from a new, deeper tone to a high-pitched squeak, all in the same sentence. Under the influence of testosterone, the larynx (or voice box) undergoes structural changes. As it becomes larger, the vocal chords become longer. (The larger the larynx becomes, the deeper the voice.) The larynx cartilage (or Adam's apple) also enlarges, and because the vocal chords are stretching behind it, it gets pushed out and becomes more noticeable. All these changes combine to cause sporadic (and often unexpected!) squeaks in a boy's voice as it gradually deep-

> *"Girls are always running through my mind. They don't dare walk."*
>
> —Andy Gibb

ens. Don't worry. Most boys complete their voice change by sixteen years of age.

Going . . . Going . . . Gone!

By late puberty, facial hair is well established. For most guys, daily shaving is the norm. Pubic hair now covers the symphysis pubis (or pubic mound) and has spread to the inside thighs. Chest and leg hair is denser, and for some young men, shoulder and back hair have emerged, too.

Although "late bloomers" may still be growing, most guys reach adult height by age seventeen. However, that doesn't mean all growth stops. Muscle development can continue much longer, even into early adulthood.

Now for the question on every guy's mind: is that as big as it gets? For most young men, final adult penile length—which is genetically determined—is reached by puberty's end. Contrary to locker room boasts, however, a penis's "at rest" size is not indicative of its erect size, effectiveness, or masculinity. Just as women's breasts vary greatly, so do men's penises. There's a wide range of lengths and widths that are all considered normal.

By the end of puberty, the little boy is gone, replaced by a young man fully capable of reproduction. As with young women, physical ability to reproduce is not reflective of cognitive and emotional readiness in young men. Remember, psychosocial development is still lagging behind.

Hormones rage in puberty, and just as these hormones impact the physical you, they also impact the emotional you. You might experience strong emotions you've never encountered before. Or maybe you've felt overly sensitive and easily upset. Some teens lose their tempers and find themselves easily irritated with friends and family. Others cry over the slightest thing.

Now throw in sexual feelings, as if the others weren't enough. It's really difficult to deal with all these new emotions. So it's important to remember that while your body is adjusting to hormonal changes, so is your mind. It's all normal, and it will get easier. Just give yourself time. If you have any concerns about these pubertal changes, don't be afraid to talk with a trusted adult.

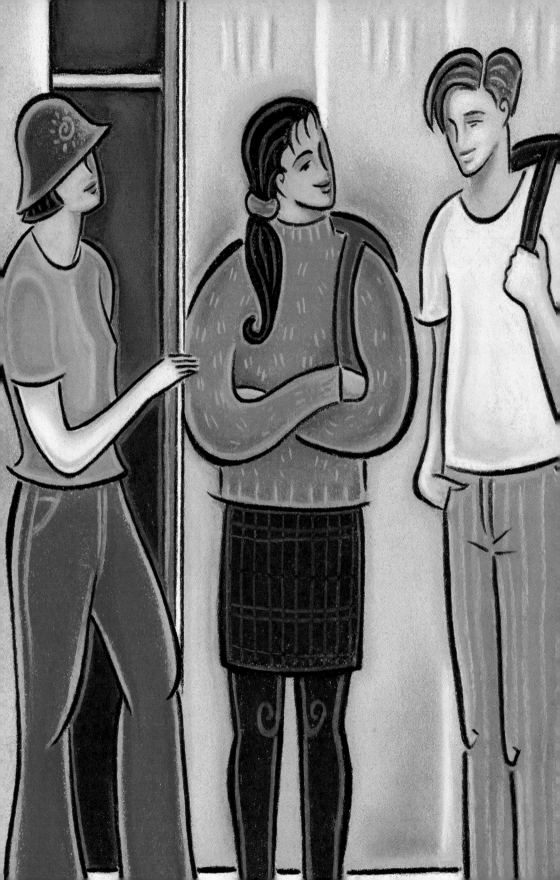

5

EXTREME TEENS:

Social Development
and Peer Pressure

In chapter 2, we
explored cognitive and
emotional development.
We also examined an off-
shoot, psychosocial development, noting four arenas
of development necessary
to maturity: individuation,
self-awareness, realistic

goal-setting, and *mature* participation in peer and intimate relationships. Because the last arena—relationships—is complex and crucial to psychosocial maturity, we're giving it its own chapter.

If you recall, psychosocial development usually emerges over three, distinct adolescent stages: early adolescence, middle adolescence, and late adolescence. What do teens socially look like in each stage?

Bianca has become painfully aware of *every*thing. She's self-conscious about her family, her beliefs, her house, her parents' car, her clothes, her backpack (not to mention what's in it), her hair, her skin, her make-up, her emerging breasts and widening hips, her height and weight, her breath and body odor, and even what she says and how she says it. Once an outgoing little girl, she

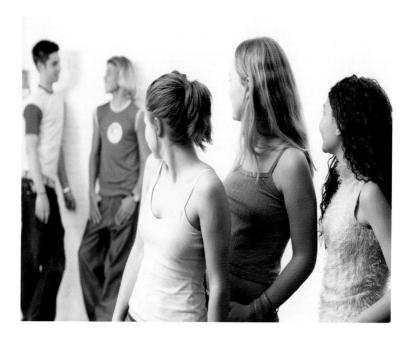

> *"The only normal people are the ones you don't know well!"*
>
> —Joe Ancis

is plagued with shyness now. *Who AM I?* she wonders. Looking at the crowd of girls she longs to join, she shakes her head. *Will I ever fit in?*

Early Adolescent Relationships (Ages Ten to Thirteen)

Friends

For the first time since birth, this age group now prefers spending time with friends over family. Single-sex groups are the norm. Girls are more relational in these groups, while boys tend to interact more physically. If you watch preteens on any playground, chances are you'll find clusters of girls scattered across the yard, gossiping in huddles, while boys are likely shooting hoops, pushing and shoving, or kicking a soccer ball.

In this stage, appearances mean everything. These kids go to great lengths to "fit in." Clothing, hairstyles, make-up, piercing, brand names—nothing seems to be off-limits in the pursuit of acceptance. Like Bianca's, insecurities flourish. Peer pressure is enormous, and many

Piercing the Pack: Surviving the Clique Mentality

1. Expand your circle of friends. Don't limit yourself. Be part of other groups.
2. Make decisions that are yours alone, despite what anyone says or does.
3. Be true to your moral convictions. Resist peer pressure when it counts! (Pressuring you to see a movie is one thing; pressuring you into crime, drugs or sex is quite another. "Friends" who do are not friends at all.)
4. Form your own opinions. And SPEAK them. (Standing up for what you believe is an important milestone in psychosocial development and a sign of maturity.)
5. Suggest something new to do. If your group dismisses the idea or even laughs at you, do it anyway with someone else!

"early ads" find security in looking like those around them. Familiar ground feels comfortable and safe.

Because individuation is incomplete, most early adolescents search for their identity in groups, rather than within. "Blending in" offers **anonymity**, not to mention a momentary and welcome reprieve from self. A popular illusion is that everyone *else* has it together. (That holds true only until you get to know the other person!)

Besides, mimicking is easy—certainly a lot less taxing than creating a new you, particularly when, as yet, most lack the necessary psychological skills and maturity to do so. Hanging out with others, copying what they say and what they wear, can actually become a haven in the storm of self-discovery. In a sense, you can avoid yourself.

Sadly, though, for a few teens, that's not enough. Some early adolescents not only gravitate toward those like them, they also tend to move away from, **ostracize**, and poke fun at anyone who's not. **Cliques** abound. **Exclusivity**, taunts, and teasing are widespread. For these reasons, this stage is perhaps the cruelest of the adolescent stages.

Try to remember that no matter how tempting it is, you should never have to look, act, dress, or think like anyone else to fit in. Your likes, what you believe, how you think—these are the things that make you special, the one and only you. What truly matters are things that can't be measured from the outside.

Beating a Bully: Five Survival Tips

1. If you're in physical danger, tell a trusted adult. Your safety comes first.
2. Avoid being alone. Stick close to friends. Think: group survival!
3. Ignore it. Walk away. (It takes more courage NOT to reply.) The message you send is that you don't care, and he or she will eventually get bored of picking on someone who doesn't respond.
4. Use body language. Keep your head up. Act confident. You want to convey that you're neither scared nor vulnerable, just indifferent.
5. Try humor. If you agree and laugh at yourself, you won't give the bully the satisfaction of the response he or she was trying to get out of you.

More Than Friends

For the young end of the bracket (preteens ages ten and eleven), relating with the opposite sex is, at best, awkward and, at worst, "icky." Cooties are still real! Puberty is just kicking in, so sexual concepts seem foreign, mysterious, or even disgusting.

"Check this out!" Lisa urges in a hushed voice. Four preteen girls scurry over and crowd around her older brother's dresser drawer.

"It's just a deck of cards," one observes.

"Not just *any* cards," Lisa insists. "Look."

As she fans out the deck, entwined naked bodies in various sexual positions illustrate the front of each card. Oral sex is not neglected.

"Eeeeeew. That's *gross!*" one friend squeals. "Who would do THAT?"

On the other hand, at the older end of this age bracket, some twelve- and thirteen-year-olds begin to experience and explore feelings of sexuality. At this point, though, they're working from hormones, curiosity, and limited examples set for them by parents or other close adults. Genuine understanding of relationships and sexuality is almost nonexistent. Some older "early ads" can begin to have romantic fantasies, but they will usually remain just that. These factors, coupled with a changing body and a new sense of self-awareness, often lead to intense self-consciousness and embarrassment.

Egocentricity (self-centeredness) drives the "dating" urge now. "Going out" is based on what each individual gets out of the relationship. Popularity, feeling included, entrance into a clique, a more positive self-image, companionship for an event, or simple fun can motivate relationships.

I can't believe Cara said no, Derrick broods. His friends are all going to the seventh grade winter dance. Everyone is. *I don't really know anyone else I'd like to take that's not already going. Wait a minute . . . What about Rachel? She's kinda cute . . . sort of okay. She's all right . . . and I bet she'd go.*

Derrick really isn't interested in dating. Nor is he really interested in Rachel. He just wants to go to the dance. In essence, he's looking out for himself, using Rachel to fill a social need. Such selfish motives are common at this age. Early teens lack the psychosocial maturity to mutually love.

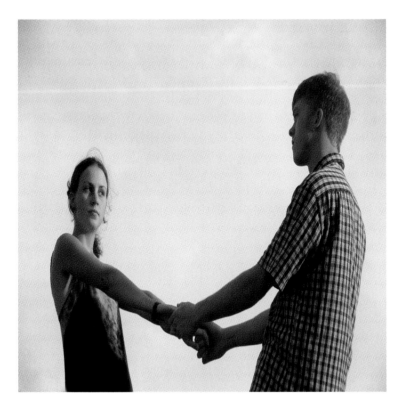

MIDDLE ADOLESCENCE (AGES FOURTEEN TO SEVENTEEN)

FRIENDS

Relationship-wise, "mid-adolescents" still favor hanging with peers over family, but their circle widens to include both sexes. Girls are definitely still into "relating" with friends (of either sex) while boys are still more into "doing." Mixed-group activities are common.

"Do you want to go to the mall Saturday?" Sara invites. Since they were thirteen, Marie and Sara have spent Saturday afternoons together at the mall, or at least in each other's bedrooms trading clothes. Now they're sixteen.

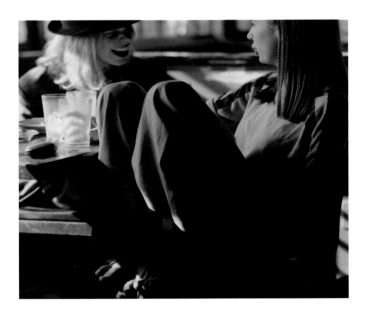

"Nah," Marie replies. "Becky, Greg, Jude, and I are mountain biking that morning, then Jude's taking me to the football game." She hesitates. "You know, I really don't like the mall that much anymore. It's sort of boring." Guilt-ridden, she quickly adds, "But maybe you could go with us to the game?"

Friendships often rearrange and change during this period. While teens are evolving into young adults, many try out new things to figure out who they are. Like Marie, maybe your best childhood friend has traded in malls for males and clothes for cycling. Maybe that old soccer teammate has exchanged cleats for cameras. Or maybe another friend has traded in laughs for love. It's all normal.

Still, when friends start to grow apart, it's hard! It can leave you feeling hurt, left out, and as though you don't matter anymore. Feelings like these are common. Remember, as friends are discovering who they are, so too are you. You're cultivating your own grown-up identity. That identity may or may not include friends from younger years. Either way, in no time, you'll be involved in new, more mature friendships that might last a lifetime. For some, they do.

More Than Friends

Teens in this age group have generally completed most of their pubertal development (see chapters 3, 4, and 5), but psychosocial abilities may not be as evolved. If you recall, psychosocial maturation can continue through young adulthood. Consequently, this stage of development is often confusing and tumultuous because the body is ahead of the mind. (See chapter 2.)

Casual dating is common, and tends to lack depth and emotional maturity. Most kids this age aren't developed

Cardiac Care for Teens: Mending a Broken Heart

Broken hearts hurt; try these tips to lessen the pain:

1. Share your feelings with someone you trust. Let them know what you're going through. Get it out. Talk about it all. Let the tears flow.
2. Keep yourself busy. Movies and books offer great escapes. Or start a project like redecorating your room. Shift your focus!
3. Remember what's good about *you*. Everyone has positive traits; you do, too. If you're too crushed to be objective, have friends over to help you see the real you.
4. Give yourself time. It takes a while—weeks, months, even years for some—for a broken heart to mend.
5. Stay healthy. Exercise. Eat right. Physically pamper yourself a bit.

enough psychosocially to grasp the unselfishness that defines mature relationships. They remain centered on themselves. "Going out" tends to be a shallow relationship—despite strong feelings—and deeply committed relationships are rare. It seems as though mid-adolescents are constantly breaking up, then dating someone new. Hearts fracture sooner than later.

Younger mid-ads tend to start dating as groups, while older mid-ads move into more one-on-one relationships. Mid-ads, like young ads, have sexual fantasies, and some begin to explore these fantasies more physically, testing out sexual behaviors with actual partners. Pressure to have sex can be huge.

"C'mon," Josh urges. "What's the problem? I'll be safe."

Josh and Anne have been dating for a few months. They've rarely had time alone, but the few chances they've had led to some kissing, fondling, and foreplay. Josh thinks he's ready for intercourse.

Anne is hesitant. She really likes Josh, and she wants him to like her, too. *I'm so confused*, she silently acknowledges. *I don't know what to do!* Anne would do just about anything to please or impress Josh, but emotionally she isn't ready for intercourse. *All these feelings . . .* Her body does respond to his touch, and she enjoys every sensation. *It would be so easy to just say yes . . . so tempting.* She admits she likes Josh, but does she love him? Honestly, she can't say. She really wants her first time to be with that special person she'll love forever. *Josh is definitely not the one, but how can I say no and not lose him?*

Abstinence Is a Choice: Why Some Teens Wait

1. pregnancy prevention (It's the most effective form of birth control!)
2. protection against STDs (Some STDs like AIDS make the decision to have sex a life-or-death situation, and many teens take that seriously.)
3. strong moral convictions
4. religious beliefs
5. self-knowledge/self-respect: knowing they're just not ready and honoring that

---

Seven Signs of a Healthy Relationship

(These can be applied to both friendships and romantic relationships.)

1. equality: mutual give-and-take (not one-sided giving or taking)
2. mutual respect: valuing the person without trying to change him or her
3. honesty
4. trust: honoring the relationship's privacy and encouraging its dependability
5. individual identities: the freedom to be who you each are and to pursue new ideas, interests and friends
6. unconditional support: a shoulder to cry on AND hands to applaud
7. regular, clear, immediate, and tactful communication

No one likes to feel inferior or left out. Everyone wants and needs to be liked. We all long for approval. Sadly, many middle adolescents mistakenly think sex is the ticket to being liked. Additionally, hormones are raging by now. Sexual sensations and thoughts can't be denied. Such feelings are nothing to feel ashamed or embarrassed about. They're perfectly healthy, indicating that sexual development (puberty) is progressing normally.

Sometimes feelings, compounded by curiosity, lead a mid-teen to thinking it's the right time to have sex when it's really not. These are powerful feelings! Don't under estimate them. You may also feel pressured by a date to

Red Flags: Eight Indications Your Relationship
Might Be Headed for Violence

1. Seeing respective friends is off limits.
2. Interacting with the opposite sex, no matter how innocently, is off limits, and can trigger outbursts of jealousy and anger.
3. Cutting a partner off from his or her family.
4. Public ridicule (making fun of job, intelligence, looks, etc.).
5. Forcing one to give up something they love, despite how much they love it.
6. Telling a partner, "Who would want you?"
7. Other forms of violence: punching a wall, throwing things, etc.
8. Intense control of everything: clothing, phone calls, interactions, activities, etc.

spected. It's no longer as important to conform, although shared established interests usually draw clusters of friends together (for example, the outdoors, the arts, areas of study, etc.). Friendships continue to rearrange as college and work-related friends often displace high-school friends. Many friendships secured at this stage will remain well into adulthood, even for life.

More Than Friends

By the end of this stage, healthy late-adolescents should be able to enter an intimate relationship offering as much as they expect to receive. This kind of mutual give-and-take is the hallmark of mature, adult relationships.

Right On Schedule

(Some late-adolescents enter adulthood never achieving this milestone of psychosocial maturity. Sadly, they're destined to leave a lonely trail of hurt in their wake.)

Sexual behavior now includes physical intimacy and frequently, intercourse. As mutual respect increases, not to mention self-respect, outside pressure to have sex wanes, although it can still be an issue. Such pressure reveals relational immaturity and can be a red flag to later abusive behavior. If sexually active, safe sex practices become a must! (Please see chapter 6.)

Peer Pressure and Its Consequences

Peer pressure takes various forms and can lead to considering—even doing—the craziest things. We all know the obvious ones: smoking, drinking, drugs, driving under the influence. But there are other, just as lethal behaviors adolescents adopt for the sake of fitting in.

Shoplifting

Some teens will shoplift (risking criminal prosecution, destroyed college plans, fines, and even jail time) just to prove that they can fit in with "cool" friends who also steal. Maybe they're answering a dare, or maybe they don't have enough money to buy the same, expensive clothes they see on classmates. Either way, they become losers to impress losers. Unfortunately, it's more common than you think.

Plastic Surgery

We're speaking here of *cosmetic* procedures that alter a part of the body a person is unhappy with. We are not talking about medically recommended, ***reconstructive surgery*** for birth defects and traumatic injuries or disease. We are also not addressing the teen whose living is genuinely inhibited by a truly outstanding feature. No, we are addressing the teen who, just because someone made a remark about her breast size, decides to have implants (augmentation mammoplasty) or breast reduction (reduction mammoplasty) to please the masses. Whatever the body part or procedure, this type of reaction to peer pressure is extreme.

If you feel compelled to have cosmetic surgery, particularly as a result of peer pressure, you need to discuss it at length with your parents and doctor. You also might want to consider these facts before committing to invasive surgery:

- The human body continues to grow into young adulthood. Breasts or noses that appear disproportionate now might become proportionate in time. Give yourself a few years!
- ALL teens are self-conscious about their bodies. Much of your self-consciousness will fade.
- Emotions have a huge effect on how you perceive yourself. If the root of your dissatisfaction is emotional (like clinical depression), merely changing a physical trait won't solve anything. Treat the emotions first, then re-evaluate. You might be surprised.

Fascinating Facts

- According to the U.S. Census Bureau, teens ages thirteen to seventeen make up just seven percent of the U.S. population, but they account for nearly thirty percent of all arrested shoplifters.
- In the United States, shoplifters steal about $25 million in merchandise daily.
- According to the American Society of Plastic Surgeons, in the year 2000, 306,384 patients eighteen years old or younger had some form of cosmetic surgery, making up four percent of the 7.4 million cosmetic surgeries performed that year. (Excludes reconstructive surgery.)
- In a National Institute on Drug Abuse (NIDA) 1999 survey, researchers found that 2.7 percent of eighth and tenth graders and 2.9 percent of twelfth graders reported anabolic steroid use at least once in their lives.
- According to a U.S. Secret Service investigation of forty-one school shooters involved in thirty-seven incidents, two-thirds of the shooters described being persecuted or bullied by their peers.

- Getting in good shape can alter a person's looks without needing surgery.

STEROIDS

Some teens, particularly guys, fall into the trap of thinking they can only be handsome or tough if they're muscularly defined and massive. Remember our discussion of body types? Some somatotypes aren't designed to be bulky, and these types of bodies resist muscle-building. Others are just lean and lanky. Some boys mature more slowly and are plagued by boy-like bodies until mid- or late-adolescence. Unfortunately, seeing more muscular bodies in the locker room sometimes drives teens to steroid use, so they too can bulk up or hurry physical maturity along. That's dangerous.

Steroids are addictive drugs. Because they affect hormonal levels, they can also affect mood and personality. Long-term use often leads to aggressive, violent behavior or paranoia, confusion, and obsessive tendencies. Steroids can also shrink boys' testicles and make girls appear more masculine. Yes, these chemicals will bulk up your muscles, but young men have also been known to become physically abusive or committed suicide while using steroids. No amount of peer pressure is worth that.

We'll talk more about other health and safety issues in our next chapter.

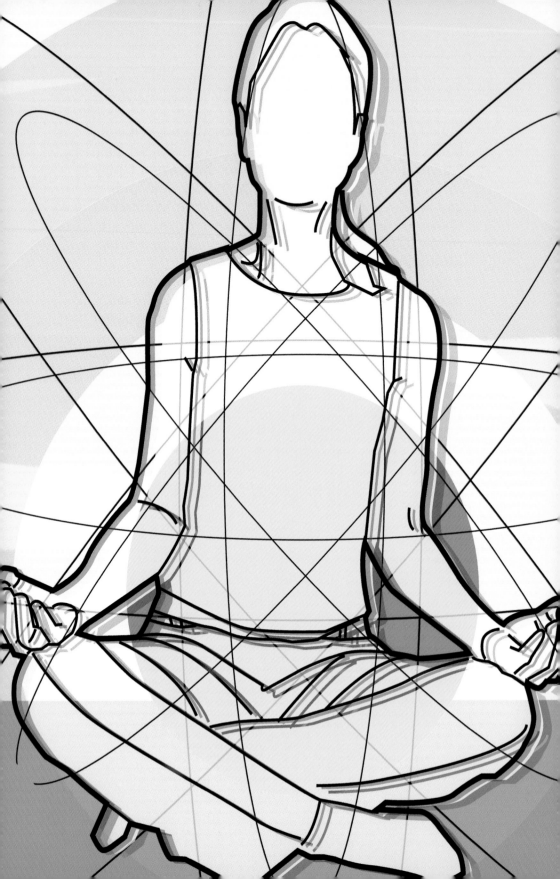

6

EXTREME CARE:

Staying Healthy and Safe

Brian, Mark, Chas, Stephanie, and Maryanne walked to the door. No one spoke a word. They didn't have to; they knew each other's thoughts. These five had experienced every "first" together since childhood.

Death was just one more.

"I can't believe he'd kill himself," Chas choked out, but it could have been any of them. They all thought the same thing.

Don't let anyone try to kid you. The adolescent years are hard years, perhaps the hardest. Ask any adult if they'd go back. Chances are you'll hear, "No way!" Why? It's just too difficult emotionally, physically, and socially.

You've seen the fall-out. Depression, anorexia, self-mutilation, bullying, runaways, substance abuse, sexual abuse, crime, and, as the five friends described above discovered, even suicide. As an adolescent, it is critical that you stay healthy and safe.

> *"If you don't take care of your body, where will you live?"*
>
> —Unknown

In this book, we've covered six main areas of teen development: physical, cognitive, emotional, pubertal, sexual, and social. In this chapter, we'll take another look at them, this time examining health and safety concerns relevant to each.

PHYSICAL DEVELOPMENT

As we discussed in chapter 1, the key to physical health is working with your body type. Increased muscle tone, less body fat, a healthy BMI—all are possible for every type. The key is to eat right and get plenty of exercise.

Most doctors recommend that teens get some form of *aerobic* exercise for at least thirty minutes, five times a week. If you play a sport that involves running or swimming, you've got it covered. But if you don't play team sports, there are plenty of other ways to get aerobic exercise: biking, walking, jogging, swimming, line dancing, in-line skating, skiing, hiking, aerobics classes; the list is nearly endless. The key is to keep moving!

As far as eating habits, go with "everything in moderation!" No one food is evil, but there are certainly foods that are better and worse for you. Try to balance them. Limit sugars and fats, but don't eliminate them. Your body needs small quantities of each to function. Beware fads that cut entire food groups. Most important, eat a well-balanced diet keeping within ideal, daily calorie guidelines for your age and body type. (Your doctor can recommend a healthy count if you're wondering.)

Last, drink at least six to eight glasses of water a day. It's not only wonderful for the body; it's fabulous for your skin!

Cognitive Development

As the adolescent mind begins to think more like an adult's, cognitive stimulation is a must. Engage in lively but respectful debates. Ask questions. Question everything. Read about others' ideas and beliefs. Explore your own. Join a debate team, or mock trial. Trade logic puzzles with friends. All of these tasks challenge the abstract mind. Don't neglect your brain!

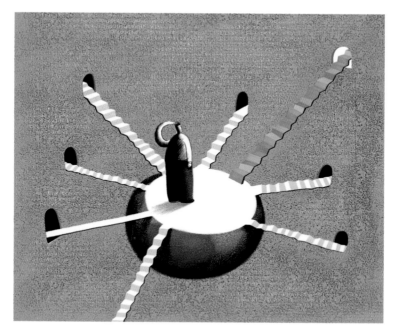

Choosing which path to take is just one of the stresses teens face.

EMOTIONAL DEVELOPMENT

What can you do to protect yourself from emotional extremes?

- Accept yourself. Learn to focus on what you like about you.
- Get plenty of rest, at least nine hours a night.
- Avoid stimulants like caffeine.
- Recognize your triggers and avoid them. (If you know a particular person really gets you upset, then keep your distance.)
- Know your cycles. If you're a girl, and you know you're irritable around ovulation, then

be alert. Recognize the cause for what it really is: hormones.

- Make time for that which soothes and relaxes
  you. Make it a priority.
- Speak your mind honestly, even hurts and
  frustrations, but with self-control and respect. If you let things bottle up, they'll ex-
  plode.
- Exercise to relieve stress.
- Pamper yourself once in a while.
- TALK ABOUT IT! Share your feelings with a
  trusted someone.
- If you notice a friend seems down, with-
  drawn, or off, gently pry. You may save a life.

General Pubertal Development

Just one recommendation can encourage health in all
but two of the areas we discussed in chapter 3: shower or
bathe daily. Keeping your body clean really will impact
the overall health of your skin and hair while eliminating
most body odor issues. As far as teeth go, brush at least
twice a day with a fluoride toothpaste.

But keeping clean won't keep you rested.

Andy has been running all day. He worked the late shift
last night, came home, caught five hours sleep, then ran
off to classes. After his last class, he drove back to work
another eight-hour shift. Now it's eleven in the evening,
and he's heading home, but first he's going to drop Ray at
his house.

Right On Schedule

"Watch out!" Ray screams. Andy jerks alert, realizing he had started to drift off. There in front of them are the headlights of an oncoming vehicle.

Not getting enough sleep can be dangerous. Rearranging your schedule to get nine hours sleep should be a priority. Your body needs the sleep! If you know that you have to get up for school by six every morning, then force yourself to be in bed by nine on weekdays, no matter how childish that might seem. If you can't, then let yourself sleep late on the weekends to make up the deficit. And if you're tired, DON'T DRIVE.

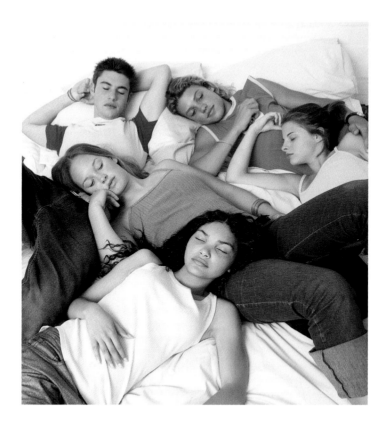

Female Puberty

Most of what needed to be said was covered in chapter 4. Two additional notes:

- Every sexually mature woman needs to start seeing a ***gynecologist*** or other health care provider annually once she's sexually active. Regular breast examinations (for precancerous growths) and annual PAP smears (screening for ***cervical*** cancer) become a must. Both breast cancer and cervical cancer are highly treatable if caught in the early stages. Annual screenings make early detection possible. Have your gynecologist teach you how to perform breast self-examinations. Then do them monthly when showering.
- Hygiene during your period is critical. Wash areas around your vagina daily. Change pads and tampons every four to six hours. These steps will help minimize infection or odor.

Male Puberty

Again, most hygiene issues like shaving and skin care were handled in earlier chapters. But young men should also be sure to have annual check-ups with their health care provider. Regular exams of the testicles, like breast exams for women, are important. Most medical practitioners handle these routine exams.

PEER PRESSURE

This area is probably the area of greatest concern when it comes to staying healthy and safe.

- Teens age fifteen to nineteen have a much higher mortality rate than younger children.
- The leading causes of death for teens are motor vehicle crashes, injury-related deaths (like from extreme sports), homicide and suicide.
- Sixty-one percent of students in grades nine through twelve reported having sexual intercourse by grade twelve.
- Fourteen percent had more than four sex partners.
- Only about half used a condom the last time they had sex.
- In 2001, 4,428 cases of **HIV** among teens thirteen to nineteen were reported in the United States.

If you think peer pressure has nothing to do with these facts, you're misguided. Sometimes, teens just don't think. Others are dealing with bodies that are light years ahead of their minds. Whatever the causes, caution is the name of the game.

Don't let anyone manipulate you into doing anything you're uncomfortable with. They're not worth it—and you *are* worth the embarrassment of saying no. Take pride in who you are, and stand up for what you believe. Be true to your convictions; there's no better sign of social maturity.

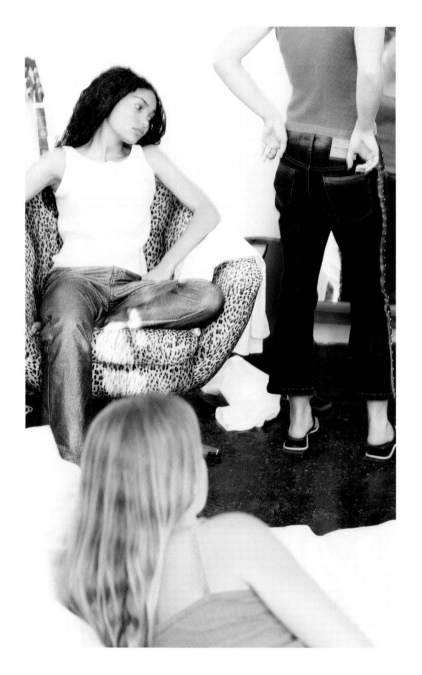

Right On Schedule

Here are some tips to keep you safe:

- Trusted friends are perhaps one of the best weapons against poor judgment. Surround yourself with wise people. If you know there's a friend with whom you get a bit crazy, make sure you invite at least one levelheaded friend to join the two of you.
- If you find yourself in a sticky situation, it's never too late to turn back. Minimize the damage, retreat and move on.
- Learn from past errors (don't pretend they didn't happen)
- NEVER DRINK AND DRIVE
- Never take the wheel when you're sleepy

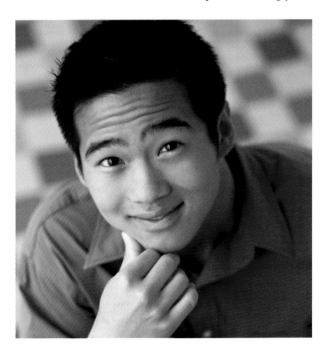

- Remember: there's safety in numbers. (This is particularly true for young women. Don't go anywhere alone with anyone you don't know quite well. Most women are raped by acquaintances.)
- Never accept a poured or open drink (even a glass of soda) from someone you don't know well.
- If you choose to have sex, practice safe sex. Talk with your doctor or parents about safe sex methods and birth control.
- Don't minimize how much help adults can be. Seek one out, especially if you feel you or a friend are in trouble.

If you're reading this book, then you're clearly interested in what's best for you. Knowledge is half that battle. You're halfway there! But knowledge left idle can't help you become that extreme teen. In order to be the best "one-and-only-you," you have to *do* some things as well. That's up to you.

FURTHER READING

GENERAL DEVELOPMENT

American Academy of Child and Adolescent Psychiatry. *Your Adolescent: Emotional, Behavioral, and Cognitive Development from Early Adolescence through the Teen Years.* New York: HarperCollins, 1999.

Bell, Ruth. *Changing Bodies, Changing Lives.* New York: Times Books, 1998.

Carnegie Council on Adolescent Development. *Great Transitions: Preparing Adolescents for a New Century.* New York: Carnegie Corporation of New York, 1995.

McCoy, Kathy. *The New Teenage Body.* New York: Putnam, 1992.

World Book, Inc. *World Book's Managing Your Teenage Life.* Chicago: World Book, 2003.

ON GIRLS

Frankenberger, Elizabeth. *Crushes, Creeps and Classmates: A Girl's Guide to Getting Along with Boys.* New York: Rosen, 1999.

Kahaner, Ellen. *Everything You Need to Know about Growing Up Female.* New York: Rosen, 1997.

Snyderman, Dr. Nancy L. *Girl in the Mirror: Mothers and Daughters in the Years of Adolescence.* New York: Hyperion, 2002.

ON BOYS

Akagi, Cynthia G. *Dear Michael: Sexual Education for Boys Ages 11-17*. Littleton, Colo.: Gylantic Publishing Company, 1996.

Felig, Paul. *Kick Me: Adventures in Adolescence*. New York: Three Rivers Press, 2002.

TEEN ISSUES

Evans, Patricia. *Teen Torment: Overcoming Verbal Abuse*. Avon, Mass.: Adams Media Corporation, 2003.

Field, Lynda. *The Self-Esteem Workbook: An Interactive Approach to Changing Your Life*. Rockport, Mass.: Element, 1995.

Garbarino, James. *And Words Can Hurt Forever: How to Protect Adolescents from Bullying, Harassment, and Emotional Violence*. New York: Free Press, 2002.

Holyoke, Nancy. *A Smart Girl's Guide to Boys: Surviving Crushes, Staying True to Yourself and Other Love Stuff*. Middleton, Wisc.: American Girl, 2001.

Lang, Denise. *But Everyone Else Looks So Sure of Themselves: A Guide to Surviving the Teen Years*. White Hall, Ver.: Shoe Tree Press, 1991.

McCoy, Kathy. *Life Happens: A Teenager's Guide to Friends, Failure, Rejection, Addiction, Peer Pressure, Families, Loss, Depression, Change, and Other Challenges of Living*. New York: Berkley Publishing Group, 1996.

Packer, Alex J. *Highs!: Over 150 Ways to Feel Really, Really Good . . . without Alcohol or Other Drugs.* Minneapolis: Free Spirit Publishing, 2000.

Shandler, Sara. *Ophelia Speaks: Adolescent Girls Write about Their Search for Self.* Thorndike, Me.: Thorndike Press, 2000.

Vandenburg, Mary Lou. *Coping with Being Shy.* New York: Rosen, 1993.

Young, Bettie B. *A Taste-Berry Teen's Guide to Setting and Achieving Goals: With Contributions by Teens for Teens.* Deerfield Beach, Fla.: Health Communications, 2002.

American Academy of Child and Adolescent Psychiatry
www.aacap.org/

American Medical Association
www.ama-assn.org/ama/pub/category/1981.html (Adolescent Health Page)

Center for Young Women's Health,
Children's Hospital, Boston
www.youngwomenshealth.org

Cool Nurse
www.coolnurse.healthology.com

Keep Kids Healthy
www.keepkidshealthy.com

Kids' Health
www.kidshealth.org.
www.kidshealth.org/teen/your_body

National Centers for Disease Control and Prevention (or CDC) - Adolescent Health page with links
www.cdc.gov/node.do/id/0900f3ec801e457a

National Institute of Child Health and Development
www.nichd.nih.gov

National Institutes of Health
health.nih.gov/result.asp/657/24

National Institute of Mental Health
www.nimh.nih.gov

National Library of Medicine
www.nlm.nih.gov

Palo Alto Medical Foundation
www.pamf.org/teens
www.pamf.org/teen/parents/health/growth-11-14.html
www.pamf.org/teen/parents/health/growth-15-17.html

Science Education Partnerships
www.seps.org
www.pearlsforteengirls.com

Teen Growth
www.teengrowth.com

Teen Health Centre
www.teenhealthcentre.com

Wired for Youth
www.wiredforyouth.com/health.cfm

Publisher's note:
The Web sites listed on these pages were active at the time of publication. The publisher is not responsible for Web sites that have
changed their addresses or discontinued operation since the date of
publication. The publisher will review and update the Web sites
upon each reprint.

abstinent Voluntarily holding back.

aerobic Living, active, or occurring only in the presence of oxygen.

anemia A condition in which the blood is deficient in red blood cells, in hemoglobin, or in total volume.

anonymity (an-oh-NIM-it-ee) The quality or state of being unnamed or unidentified.

asynchrony (a-SIN-crow-nee) The condition of not occurring at the same time.

causal relationships Relationships expressing or indicating a reason for an action or condition.

cellulite Lumpy fat found in the thighs, hips, and buttocks of some women.

cervical Of or relating to the cervix, the narrow outer end of the uterus.

chronic Marked by long duration or frequent recurrence; not acute.

circadian (sir-CAY-dee-en) Occurring in approximately 24-hour periods or cycles.

cliques (clicks) Narrow or exclusive circles or groups of people.

clitoris (cli-TOR-us) A small erectile organ at the front of the female vulva.

cognitively Having to do with awareness and judgment.

cosmetic Of, relating to, or making for beauty, especially of the complexion.

deciduous (dee-SID-joo-us) Falling off or shed seasonally or at a certain stage of development in the life cycle.

dermatologist A medical doctor who specializes in the skin, its structure, functions, and diseases.

dominant Of, relating to, or exerting ecological or genetic influence or control.

exclusivity The state of being limited to possession, control, or use by a single individual or group.

hypotheses Assumptions or guesses made for the sake of argument.

incremental Increasing, especially in quantity or value.

individuation (in-di-vid-JOO-ay-shun) The act or process of forming into a separate person.

intangible Not capable of being perceived, especially by the sense of touch.

genes The packages of hereditary information on a chromosome.

gynecologist (gine-uh-COL-o-jist) A medical doctor who specializes in the diseases and routine physical care of the reproductive system of women.

HIV Human immunodeficiency viruses are any of a group of retroviruses that infect and destroy helper T cells of the immune system.

labia (LAY-bee-uh) Folds at the margin of the vulva.

metabolic (met-uh-BOL-ik) Of, relating to, or based on metabolism, the chemical changes in living cells by which energy is provided for vital processes and activities and new material is absorbed.

orthodontist A dentist who specializes in irregularities of the teeth and their correction (as by means of braces).

ostracize Exclude by general consent from common privileges or social acceptance.

ovaries Female reproductive organs that produce eggs.

pituitary gland (pi-TWO-i-terry) A small endocrine organ attached to part of the brain that produces various internal secretions directly or indirectly affecting most basic body functions.

plaque (plack) A film of mucous that harbors bacteria on a tooth.

precocious (pruh-COH-shus) Exceptionally early in development or occurrence.

psychosocially In a way that involves both psychological and social aspects.

pubertal (PU-ber-tul) Of or relating to puberty, the condition of being or the period of becoming first capable of reproducing sexually.

reconstructive surgery Surgery to restore function or normal appearance by remaking defective organs or parts.

relativity The quality or state of not being absolute or definite.

repertoire (rep-er-TWAR) A list or supply of capabilities.

recessive A gene that does not express its instructions when paired with a dominant gene.

scrotum The external pouch that contains the testes.

somatotypes (so-MAT-oh-types) Body types; physiques.

synchrony (sin-CROW-nee) Occurrence, arrangement, or treatment at precisely the same time.

tactile Perceptible by touch.

testes Male reproductive glands that produce sperm.

testicles Testes, usually with their enclosing structures.

uterus An organ of the female mammal for containing and usually for nourishing the young during development previous to birth; womb.

vagina A canal in a female mammal that leads from the uterus to the external orifice of the genital canal.

INDEX

PICTURE CREDITS

Corbis pp. 61, 62
Eyewire pp. 10, 28, 48, 81, 86
iDream p. 30, 66, 110
Image Source pp. 32, 51, 88, 112, 115
LifeART pp. 77, 79
National Center for Health Statistics pp. 18, 19, 21,
    22
Photos.com pp. 93, 99
Photodisc pp. 14, 27, 37, 40, 58, 68, 74, 94, 106, 116

The individuals in these photographs are models,
    and the images are for illustrative purposes only.

Jean Ford is a freelance author, writer, illustrator, and public speaker. She resides in Perkasie, Pennsylvania, with her husband of twenty years, Michael, and their two adolescent children Kristin and Kyle. Her work is international, as she writes for periodicals from the United States to China, and speaks to audiences as far away as Africa. Although she generally writes adult nonfiction, she loves writing and illustrating children's books; *I Wonder: My World* is her first children's book.

Dr. Sara Forman graduated from Barnard College and Harvard Medical School. She completed her residency in Pediatrics at Children's Hospital of Philadelphia and a fellowship in Adolescent Medicine at Children's Hospital Boston (CHB). She currently is an attending in Adolescent Medicine at CHB, where she has served as Director of the Adolescent Outpatient Eating Disorders Program for the past nine years. She has also consulted for the National Eating Disorder Screening Project on their high school initiative and has presented at many conferences about teens and eating disorders. In addition to her clinical and administrative roles in the Eating Disorders Program, Dr. Forman teaches medical students and residents and coordinates the Adolescent Medicine rotation at CHB. Dr. Forman sees primary care adolescent patients in the Adolescent Clinic at CHB, at Bentley College, and at the Germaine Lawrence School, a residential school for emotionally disturbed teenage girls.